PASTORAL RESPONSES
TO SEXUAL ISSUES

Other Westminster/John Knox Press Books
by William V. Arnold

Introduction to Pastoral Care

Christians and the Art of Caring

When You Are Alone

PASTORAL RESPONSES TO SEXUAL ISSUES

William V. Arnold

Westminster/John Knox Press
Louisville, Kentucky

Scripture quotations from the New Revised Standard Version of the Bible are copyright © 1989 by the Division of Christian Education of the National Council of the Churches of Christ in the U.S.A., and are used by permission.

Book design by Carol Dukes Eberhart

First Edition

Published by Westminster/John Knox Press
Louisville, Kentucky

This book is printed on acid-free paper that meets the American National Standards Institute Z39.48 standard. ∞

PRINTED IN THE UNITED STATES OF AMERICA

9 8 7 6 5 4 3 2 1

Library of Congress Cataloging-in-Publication Data

Arnold, William V.
   Pastoral Responses to Sexual Issues / William V. Arnold.
       p.   cm.
   Includes bibliographical references.
   ISBN 0–664–25450–0 (alk. paper)
     1. Pastoral counseling.   2. Sex—Religious aspects—Christianity.
3. Sexual ethics.   4. Sex counseling.   I. Title.
BV4012.2.A75   1993
259'.08'69—dc20   93–10750

This book is dedicated to my wife,
Margaret Anne,
with whom I have coauthored two books.
We had hoped to make this book a joint project,
but her responsibilities at the church made it impossible.
Nonetheless, she has made helpful suggestions throughout
and enjoyed "editing" my work as much as ever!
Her person and her sensitivity are gifts to me,
and the readers of this book are beneficiaries of them.

Contents

CONTENTS

Acknowledgments

More people contribute to the writing of a book than even the author knows. Nonetheless, I want to list those of whom I am particularly conscious.

This work began in earnest during my sabbatical year in 1991. President T. Hartley Hall IV and Dean of Faculty Charles M. Swezey not only made provision for the time, according to seminary policy, but they were also encouraging and supportive beyond what is expected.

I spent the year away from the campus of Union Theological Seminary in Virginia, where I teach, and lived in Bryn Mawr, Pennsylvania, where my wife, Margaret Anne Fohl, serves as one of the pastors of the Bryn Mawr Presbyterian Church. That staff and that congregation received me into their midst and sensitively offered a delicate balance of welcoming me, inviting me to participate and teach from time to time in the life of the church, and affording me privacy to pursue my study and writing.

During that year in the Philadelphia area, I had the opportunity to spend time reading and taking classes at the Marriage Council of Philadelphia. Both faculty and support staff were cordial and helpful. In particular, I appreciated Steve Treat's helping me decide how to take best advantage of my time there, Gerald Weeks's careful attention to the variety of perspectives available to a person working with relational issues, and Larry Hof's breadth of knowledge in the arena of sexual issues. All of these people provided stimulation and helpfulness. However, I should excuse them from any culpability for my perspectives and approaches by saying that this book is not an attempt to present that institution's perspective. In the final analysis, the views are my own distillation from a variety of perspectives and experiences.

As I began to work through the early stages of the manuscript, I sought the help of pastoral counselors who possessed clinical experience and still maintained close ties with the life of the parish. I found just that in the members of the staff of Brandywine Pastoral Institute in Wilmington, Delaware. J. Thomas Ledbetter, Donna C. Strachan, and Christopher C. Schooley (a former student of mine) met with me on several occasions to review at length my perspectives and my ability to communicate technical material in a readable way for parish pastors. Though I had to return to Richmond before the completion of the book, I am grateful for their help in orienting me more clearly in the beginning.

Ruthanne Schlarbaum, a member of the Bryn Mawr church, a writer herself, and the daughter of a Presbyterian pastor, helped me immensely by reading the manuscript from the perspectives of both writer and churchperson. Because of her sensitivity to the nuances of language and communication, my expression is clearer.

This is the third book that has brought with it the opportunity to work with editor Harold Twiss. His thoroughness never ceases to amaze me, as well as the gentle way in which he can ask questions that reveal important opportunities to be more thorough and clear. For his insightful "shepherding" of me through the avenues of publication, I am more than grateful.

Introduction

Sexuality is a big deal! Why? Many a pastor has probably asked that question. Sometimes blatantly, more often fearfully, some parishioners will attempt to talk directly about sexual issues with a pastor. Whether they describe their "presenting problem" as sexual or not, if an opening is provided, they will test the waters. The subject of sex will come up or at least be referred to obliquely. However, far more people will never verbalize their concern and suffer silently.

Do not exclude the pastor herself or himself from the silent group. Often, a major component of the "big deal" is the pastor's own past or current sexual experience. That personal history strongly influences the degree of willingness or reluctance to enter into conversations at a personal level about sexual issues.

The subject of sex is scary to many people in our day. Witness the extreme reactions and assertions that occur in regard to public statements on the topic. People are angry, fearful, ashamed, outraged, confused, and anxious. Yet, behind the scenes of public debates, some parishioners and nonparishioners alike come to the privacy and presumed safety of a pastor's study to ask, to confess, to agonize, to make decisions about the conduct of their lives—and those lives, more often than not, are deeply affected by sexual issues. I believe that many more would come if they could sense the pastor's own comfort with and willingness to talk about the subject.

People and families are powerfully shaped by experiences involving rape, incest, abuse, harassment, fecundity, sterility, sexual orientation, sexual satisfaction or unhappiness within marriage, birth control, abortion, extramarital sexual relationships, the AIDS crisis, gender discrimination, and a host of other related issues. There are few safe places to deal with those concerns. Yet, many women and men—single and married, children and adults, affluent and poor, young and old, able and disabled—yearn for such a "safe harbor" within which they can talk and explore and make decisions without being attacked, labeled, or shamed. And yet, in all too many cases, they are prevented from doing so by taboos or outright threats—or they do not believe that such a safe place and person exist!

Anything that functions with such power in people's lives must be close to the center of things. That is not simply a psychological statement. It is a theological one. Our sexuality is a defining element in understanding who we are and who God is. For a pastor to deal helpfully and redemptively with people, this powerful force must be made speakable and faced with courage and care.

This book is built around several affirmations. First, pastors have far more opportunities to deal with sexual issues in people's lives than they realize. Sexuality is often being dealt with in a pastoral conversation when the pastor does not even perceive it. Second, given the intensity of public debate over sexual issues, pastors must assume that there will be an increasing number of public and private occasions in which they will have opportunities to offer knowledgeable and sensitive help. Third, attempts to care will be damaging if the pastor is not aware of and open to learning more about the multiple forces that are at work in our sexuality. Fourth, the pastor's awareness must be physiological, psychological, and theological—not necessarily in that order. Sexuality is multidimensional in its content and in its effects. Fifth, the pastor cannot undertake this task strictly on the basis of intellectual information. She or he must be self-aware as well.

This book is written especially for those pastors and other caring Christians who believe in or want to explore the importance of sexual issues in ministry and who have not yet done a great deal of work in it. The book is divided into two parts.

In Part 1, the language will be more personal, inviting you into an exploration of self that centers on sexual issues and experiences. Chapter 1 will suggest a number of areas for personal reflection. It will be helpful if this early material is processed more slowly. Stop after each section of the chapter and take stock of where you are in relation to the issues raised. Whether you have engaged in such a process before or not, it is a worthwhile discipline. You will be invited to use your observations and discoveries as you read further.

Chapter 2 will broaden your introspective task by introducing more general material on sexuality and sense of self. If you have read in the field of sexuality before, you will be on familiar ground in terms of content, but the contribution of the book here is to relate the material specifically to pastoral issues. Chapter 3 addresses fundamental issues in the pastoral relationship, with particular reference to working with sexual issues. Matters of safety, personal conduct, and referral are of critical importance when dealing with sexual issues.

With Part 1 having set a tone for the pastor's general work and self-knowledge with regard to issues of sexuality, Part 2 focuses on specific sexual issues and situations that parishioners often bring to the clergy or which arise in the ongoing life of a parish. Information will be provided on ways to view the problem as well as suggestions for counsel, care, and referral when appropriate.

One criterion that "qualified" a topic for inclusion in this book was the difficulty ordinarily experienced by people in acknowledging both the problem and its resolution. For example, there could well have been a chapter on infertility, but people seem to manifest a higher level of understanding and acceptance of the pain and grief involved in that experience. There are also many well-known and encouraged options for dealing with that problem. While many people may at first feel some shame or embarrassment about their difficulty in conceiving or carrying a child to term, when another means of having children is found, there is public rejoicing.

In like manner, a chapter might have been written on sexual fears and difficulties experienced in later life. However, that topic also has been explored in much of the literature on aging.

I hope the reader will find the perspectives and suggestions discussed in this book to be of value in approaching these sexual issues as part of the larger scope of pastoral care. In the best of all worlds, genuine pastoral care will enable people to speak more openly of the things they are afraid to confront and then find choices where they have felt themselves to be powerless. While people may not find full resolution for their difficulties, at least they can have pastoral companions along the way. Then growth and understanding are more likely to occur in spite of anxiety and fear.

One further assumption of this book is that pastors are not trained, nor are they expected, to function as skilled sex therapists. Thus, this book does not attempt to so equip you. Pastors have a critical role to perform as "triage officers" on the front lines of congregational and community life. Good diagnostic ability and short-term intervention skills are vital to the welfare of a person who may need long-term therapeutic help. It is from that perspective that this book is offered as an introductory resource. Whether the public debates are settled or not, pastoral care and counseling go on. This book is devoted to the development and maintenance of that more private and vulnerable pastoral responsibility.

PART 1

THE PASTOR'S RESPONSIBILITY FOR SELF-AWARENESS

1
Caring for Others
Means Owning Up
to Who We Are

I hope that you will read this chapter in a way that is unlike your usual procedure for moving through a text. Give yourself time, as you read, to think about *yourself*. Because your own self-awareness is so critical in working with sexual issues in pastoral care, it is important to begin by bringing your own sense of self to center stage.

Living in a sexually conflicted world means—go ahead and admit it—that we are and will be conflicted as well. There are degrees of conflict, of course. Yet, if we are going to be effective in our pastoral care of others, then we must be aware and caring of ourselves as well. Therefore, this first chapter invites you to do what too many of us who do pastoral care are not comfortable in doing when we pick up a book—engaging in some *self*-examination. You can read the rest of the book, and even find it useful, without reading this first chapter. But if you take the time to engage in this reflection, you will be rewarded. If you have some personal issues in mind as you read on, you will be helped (personally and in your helping others) all the more by what is to follow. To explore your reluctance, or perhaps your eagerness, to deal pastorally with sexual issues will put you in touch with the sort of ambivalence that is going on in the minds of others as well. They, too, wonder about the cost of actually admitting the level of their concern about some sexual issue. They also wonder about the realism of hoping for resolution.

If you need even more persuasion to stay with me here, remember that John Calvin begins his *Institutes of the Christian Religion* with a section on the important connection between knowing the self and knowing God. The more we learn about God, the more we learn about the self. *And*, the more we learn about the self, the more we learn about God.

Take some notes as you go through these exercises. Later, when you look back over your work, other items of interest and importance may come into your awareness. Perhaps you might even record your thoughts on tape as you read and reflect. With only a button to push to stop and start, you might be less distracted as you pull things together in your mind. Incidentally, these exercises can also be done in a group setting, with one person slowly reading aloud the suggestions below and allowing time for reflection.

Self-Awareness

Three exercises are suggested here to help you explore memories related to your body, your family of origin, and your beliefs and values.

Exploration I: Body Memories

Take a few moments to relax. Close your eyes. Look out the window or at a soothing picture. If it's helpful, put on some music. Create an environment for yourself that will facilitate your drifting back in memory. Drift back to your earliest memories of what it was like to be a child. Remember the sounds and sights that surrounded you: voices, faces, places where you remember playing, friends you spent time with, family activities. As you remember, focus your attention on memories of *physical touches*. What do you remember that was soft and cuddly? What was hard, or cold, or even painful? Give yourself some time just to let those thoughts, feelings, and sensations flow. Then, take a few moments to write down, or at least consolidate in your memory, the ones that stand out to you.

As you recalled feelings and sensations about touch in your early life, you may have gotten in touch with images of your body. What specific memories do you have about your *body*? Concentrate more on those memories from several perspectives.

First, do you remember how you felt when *looking* at yourself in a mirror? Did you like what you saw? Did you avoid looking? When seeing yourself undressed, were you embarrassed? Curious? Delighted? Fascinated? Did you feel free to look carefully, to examine, to learn about who you were? Were feelings associated with looking at different "parts" of yourself? Record some of those memories.

Next, what do you remember about *touching* your body? Were the sensations pleasant? Or was there ambivalence? Was touching your body something done naturally and without noticing it much? Or do you remember feeling self-conscious about touch? Of course, it is important to think about whether there were *parts* of your body that attracted your attention, that you *wanted* to touch. Were there areas that gave such a sensation when touched that you both wanted and feared more physical contact? Don't assume that this reference is only to genital areas. There are many pleasurable regions in our bodies. Again, take a moment to note your observations about yourself before reading further.

Last, but certainly not least, what do you remember about the response of *other people* to you and to your body? Did your parents or significant other persons seem to like you? Did you feel valued? What did they like and not like about you? And, more specifically, what did they teach you about your body as a part of yourself? Were you encouraged to enjoy yourself? Were connections made between your worth and your appearance? Did people commend you or tease you about your body—your nose, your ears, your body shape? Were you encouraged to enjoy yourself through body contact—wrestling, hugging, squeezing, tickling? Or did such activities seem hurtful, somehow threatening? Did people seem to disapprove of your being naked or of your

showing any enjoyment or appreciation of your body? Did enjoying yourself bring approval or irritation? What effect did all these
responses from other people have on your own sense of self and
your sense of what it was to have a body that could be enjoyed?

In this arena of other people's regard for and treatment of
your body, a hard question needs to be asked. Are there memories of your body being *abused* by others or another? Abuse can
range from hitting to uncomfortable caressing or tickling to
physical stimulation of your sexual organs to physical pain
(bruises, scratches, broken bones, penetration). Have experiences
such as these been a part of the shaping of your sense of self?

We began this exercise on memory by going back to childhood, but please take a few more moments to come forward in
your history. What was it like in late childhood, adolescence, and
young adulthood for you to be an emerging self—a self with a
body that can be enjoyed and can enjoy? The issues will change,
of course. For instance, what memories from puberty do you
have about "wet dreams," masturbation, the onset of menstruation, the growth of pubic hair, the development of breasts? Are
there painful memories of incest, of being embarrassed because
of your physical development? You may want to use the questions about looking, touching, and other people's responses as
you think about these body changes.

If there are painful memories of rape or molestation, of
being "grabbed," of feeling seduced, acknowledge those events to
yourself as well.

How have those experiences of self, including your awareness
of the reactions of others, played a part in your present feelings
about yourself and, in particular, your sexuality? Are the subjects
of "body" and "sex" comfortable for you? Can you talk about
them with relative ease? Where are there conflicts for you, and
when do they seem to have originated?

If you have given yourself time to do the exercise, you have
done enough for one "session." Take some time to look back
over what you have noted and/or thought about thus far. If the

impressions and memories seem to have an organization or pattern to them, allow that insight some "space" to continue developing. Look over what you have discovered or remembered. Then, depending on your inclinations, take a walk or sit down to talk with another trusted friend or partner about what you are finding. If you choose conversation rather than solitude, do not ask for opinions at this point. Use talking to that other person as your opportunity to "sound out" and formulate what you are learning about yourself.

Remember, the purpose of this undertaking is to develop your own sensitivity to issues of sexuality. The awareness gained here, enriched by the theological exploration yet to come, is an important contributor to a genuine and willing pastoral response to those who come for conversation with us as pastors and fellow inhabitants of this sexually conflicted world.

Exploration II: Family of Origin

Professionals in the counseling field emphasize the influence of the family, particularly one's early family experience. This second self-exploration invites you to consider these family patterns as source and resource for your own levels of comfort and discomfort with sexuality.

As before, create that comfortable "space" for yourself and begin to move back in memory. This time, however, move the focus away from yourself. Instead, look at the other prominent persons in your life. Remember as much as you can about the interaction that went on among them and the things they said about each other. Ask yourself what they were teaching you indirectly about self-worth in general, and issues of closeness and distance in particular.

Intimacy has been described as the capacity genuinely to "be in your own personal space while you are also in the space you share with another" (Malone and Malone, p. 23; please see For Further Reading, below). Think about that definition as you "see" these significant people in your early life. When your father and mother were together and talking with each other, did they seem comfortable? Did one seem to "become" what the other wanted, or did one seem to become antagonistic and undesirable to the other in some way? Were they emotionally and physically close, warm, winsome, likeable in their time together? Or was there neglect, negative tension, abuse, or wariness in the air when they were in the same room? In particular, how did they touch each other? What words describe best their touching: tender, intrusive, rough, delicate, cautious, angry?

Posing these questions in terms of "either-or" extremes is not meant to imply there are only dramatic opposites. There are many shades on the continuum between these extremes. Where were they as a couple on that continuum? Did either or both of them change in some way when in the presence of the other? What was each like when away from the other? Do you remember differences?

Of course, not everyone will have both parents available in early memory. You may have been in a single-parent home, or even have been raised by others. Within that "family" context, if it was yours, look at the interaction that that parent or guardian had with others. What did you learn about his or her regard for self and others?

As you recall these memories, you may find that people other than parents or guardians are the significant persons on whom you focus. "Family" often has meant a variety of people—grandparents, teachers, special friends. Let those characters flow through your perceptions as well, and ask yourself the same questions. By their interactions and ways of relating to each other, what were they teaching about care and warmth and intimacy? What lessons were taught about the acceptability of anger and the expression of disappointment? Most important of all, what strengths and weaknesses do you still carry with you as a result of their "modeling"?

As before, take some time to record the observations and impressions that stand out to you.

Before leaving this time of concentration on family, take some time to reflect on what these important people in your life taught you about what it means to be a man or a woman *in relationship*. That, of course, is an abstract question in one sense. Yet you have learned from them some things about what is "okay" for a man to do and be and for a woman to do and be. You have also learned some things, consciously or unaware, about what is acceptable for people of different genders and of the same gender to do when with each other. For example, can men hug? Yes, you say. But, if you are a man and hug other men, does it feel forced sometimes? Are you cooperating with the modeling you received, or overruling it? If you are a woman, do you shake hands with other women when meeting? Why? What models are shaping the way you feel about such an apparently simple action? What messages do you carry with you about acceptable and unacceptable expressions of affection to family members, friends, new acquaintances, children? The answers may be simple or surprising, but they need to be very conscious. You may not have taken the time to be this specific about it before. Take the time now, and allow yourself to wonder when something seems curious.

After taking some time again to record your thoughts, look back over what you have remembered. Are there gaps? Do you have some questions about particular family members, such as grandparents or aunts and uncles? Have you found your curiosity aroused by some of what we have explored? Do you want/need to know more? That may lead you to think a bit about who in your family is a willing "historian" to give you more information on these matters.

Some people find that this sort of exploration is complex and needs to be organized carefully. A variety of techniques have been developed for doing so, including specific reflection on particular people, recording your "discoveries" and comparing them with your reflections on other family members. People who use the family-systems approach suggest constructing a genogram, their name for an emotional family tree that portrays *several* generations of one's family members. It provides a graphic presentation of the emotional characteristics found in the various family relationships. A genogram can be elaborate and calls for some "archival" research, but people often are enriched and enlightened by it. A sexual genogram is even more specific and may be of interest to you. Should you wish to pursue this course of action, suggestions for further reading about it are offered at the end of this chapter.

We have finished the second of three explorations into dimensions of yourself. Take some "time out" before we move into a final exploration.

Exploration III: Beliefs and Values

The brief journey on which we will now go is the most rational and cognitive of the three—or so it may seem. However, as you know, beliefs and values are not as rational and logical as they may at first appear. What are the beliefs and values that govern your behavior in general and your sexual behavior in particular? Those principles serve as "rules," sometimes conscious and sometimes unconscious, when you think about sex and sexuality. The origins of those rules have little to do with whether they are "true" or not. One of our goals as pastors is to identify ways to be helpful to people as they struggle with the powerful, and often conflicting, feelings associated with sex. One major source for those feelings is the values or rules that have been learned over time.

Let's begin this third exploration in a different way. Before getting too relaxed and back into memory again, take a few moments to list several of the beliefs, values, or rules that you hold with regard to sexual issues. There are several ways to go about this, such as writing, recording, or discussion with a close friend. If you choose writing, for example, you may want to just "start from scratch." Write down whatever comes to mind when you think about your most important and powerful convictions about sex and sexuality. Perhaps your list would look something like this:

1. Sexual intercourse should be restricted to marriage.
2. Homosexuality is a sin.
3. If a woman gets pregnant outside of marriage, it's her fault because she was promiscuous.

4. The church has been so rigid about sex that it has lost its influence on moral behavior.
5. Never talk about sex. Just do what comes naturally.
6. Men are by nature more interested in sex than women.

Your list may be completely different from these samples, but you get the idea. Just write down the "messages" that jump to mind when you think about rules or beliefs with regard to sexual matters.

Another approach is to design a kind of sentence-completion exercise, using items such as:

1. All men are _____.
2. All women are _____.
3. Sexual intercourse is _____.
4. Homosexuality is _____.
5. The worst sexual sin is _____.
6. Infidelity means _____.
7. _____ is unforgivable.
8. Children should be taught _____ about sex.
9. When people get older, sex should be _____.
10. When two people hug, it means _____.

Again, it is not necessary to complete these particular statements. You may prefer to make up your own. The point is that you construct an inventory of beliefs, value statements, or rules that seem to be "yours" when you think about the topic of sex.

Now, having listed your rules, move again into that relaxed state with the use of meditation, music, looking out the window, or whatever has been working for you. As you develop that comfortable environment in which your mind can feel free to roam, let yourself "wonder" about the origins of some of the beliefs and rules that you have noted.

Can you hear someone speaking to you and telling you some of these things? If so, what tone of voice delivers the instructions or invitation? Can you see someone's face when you "hear" the words? Is the face smiling, stern, concerned, anxious? Do your beliefs and rules have loving and encouraging origins? Or, are some of your sexual "instructions" associated with threats, warnings of danger, admonitions with implied punishment? Together, these memories give you a sense of the quality of comfort or discomfort that is linked to these codes for behavior that have become a part of you. For example, I know that some of my own values and beliefs grow out of experiences in which I, at an early age, heard older boys laughing and joking about the ways to take advantage of girls. There is still a sick feeling in the pit of my stomach when I think about it. That, supported by what I have learned later about harassment and outright abuse, surely has led to a hesitancy on my part about expressing physical affection unless the other person makes it clear that it is acceptable. This dynamic in me has implications for the ways in which I care for other people.

Now, in looking over your earlier list and the connections that you have made in your reflection, what patterns do you see? How do these beliefs and their associated experiences "link up" with some of the things that you have identified in the earlier explorations?

I encouraged you to make these three explorations *before* moving on with the book, because it is important to know who we are when we tackle pastoral care for people in sexual matters. Frederick Buechner says it very well in his book, *Telling Secrets*:

> Maybe nothing is more important than that we keep track, you and I, of these stories of who we are and where we have come from and the people we have met along the way because it is precisely through these stories in all their particularity, as I have long believed and often said, that God makes himself [*sic*] known to each of us most powerfully and personally. If this is true, it means that to lose track of our stories is to be profoundly impoverished not only humanly but also spiritually. (1991, p. 30)

Self-Awareness and Care for Others

In the final analysis, the focus of this book is on the care of persons experiencing ambivalence and conflict emerging from sexual feelings and actions. So, why have we begun with an emphasis on *us* instead of *them*? In addition to the fact that we *are* one of "them," there are several reasons, each of them important in pastoral care.

Protection

Self-awareness serves a protective function. The protection is both for ourselves and for the persons to whom we extend care. A theological understanding of human vulnerability and sinfulness undergirds this view.

To be human is to be limited and vulnerable to hurt. Despite our most profound wish, we are not invincible. Two responses grow naturally out of this realization that we have limitations.

First, there is a natural inclination to be alert to danger, not only against obvious and present threat but also to the perceived potential for future harm. We become vigilant out of the need to take care of ourselves.

The second response is an understandable wish that things were otherwise. Out of our yearning to be more in control of our lives than we are, we devise all kinds of ways (both consciously and unconsciously) to maintain an image of strength and to engender respect, so that people won't "mess with us." Or, on the other hand, some people exert control by manifesting weakness—hoping that "if I look pitiful enough, you won't hurt me."

Here lie some of the origins of self-deceit. Because of our discomfort with or refusal to accept human vulnerability, we are prone to deceive ourselves and to deceive others. Such a disposition does not grow necessarily out of mean motives. Rather, it is a self-deluding kind of protection based on denial of who we really are. And that is exactly what gets us into trouble. Our anxiety over our humanness, as Reinhold Niebuhr alerted us, can become the breeding ground for sin. Certainly human frailty requires that we care for ourselves and others. It would be far better if we protected ourselves through *knowing* what we face than by avoiding what we fear. But out of fear or denial, we often wind up preferring not to know.

In caring for persons experiencing sexual hurt and conflict, we are involved in some of the most painful experiences and dimensions of people's lives. We join them in wishing that some of the events and lessons they have learned just were not so. At the same time, if we are to care wisely and well, we must guard ourselves and others against creating defensive illusions and lifestyles that do even more harm—to relationships, to future ability to conceive and give birth, to work, indeed to love.

Here lies the importance of self-awareness. If we are not reasonably in control of and sensitive to our own tendencies to deceive ourselves and others, then we will *use* the people for whom we are caring. We will seek to impress them with our knowledge and expertise. We may unwittingly begin to communicate to them that we alone offer the only really trustworthy help to be found—thus casting a shadow on all of their other relationships. Or, we may so identify with them that we, knowingly or unknowingly, seduce them into caring for *us* in our pain (without our ever having to admit our need for their care). Caring conversations run the risk of becoming dominated by the caregiver's description of what he or she has been through, thus subtly supporting any silent belief in the parishioner or patient that she or he is less important than the caregiver. To the degree that we work on our self-awareness, we protect this person from becoming victim to the needs that grow out of our own human vulnerability.

Another way of developing this point is to talk about the importance and health to be found in what I call "Christian paranoia." I am a Presbyterian and thus am heavily influenced by Reformed theology. The Reformed perspective places much emphasis on our sinfulness, which includes our propensity to deceive ourselves. To have a healthy dose of this "Christian paranoia" is to be open to suspicion of ourselves and our motives.

It just is impossible, from this theological frame of reference, to be helpful to someone for purely benevolent reasons. There is always "something in it" for the giver. So as a giver, we should do our best to find out what we are getting when we are helping, and be prepared to evaluate motives and actions for the well-being of ourselves and the other person.

A great deal has appeared lately in both the media and professional literature about sexual harassment and seduction of counselees and parishioners by counselors and pastors. Such revelations are painful reminders to us of the issues discussed above. The research reveals very clearly that, more often than not, those clergy who have victimized others have been "out of touch" with their own issues and needs. They were so out of touch, in fact, that they convinced themselves that sexual involvement was a "gift," rather than seeing the harm done to the other person and the painful evidence of their own unadmitted need for nurture.

One other word, from another angle, needs to be said about protection. Protection is not just to shield the other person from us. It also has to do with protecting ourselves from them. We may well be deceived by persons who are trying to exploit us sexually. After all, to talk with someone about sex is an intimate act in itself, even if no physical contact takes place at all. People who are both fearful of and desperately in need of intimacy and affection can develop very skillful ways of attaching themselves and holding on to pastoral caregivers.

We need to be aware that our desires to be effective caregivers are, in part, protective mechanisms. The subtle belief is that if we care well, then we will be respected and thus less likely to be the victim of people who do not like us. Right? After all, we will have all of them liking us! This "helpful" pattern, however, makes us vulnerable to people who begin to control us through expressions of gratitude, extensions of special gifts, threats of disapproval or even harm if we do not give them care in the way that they want it. Without even realizing it, we can be pulled into a vortex of increasing intensity. The deeper we go, the more difficult it is to extricate ourselves. To develop our self-awareness in anticipation of dealing with such people is something like learning to be wise as serpents and innocent as doves—excellent advice from Jesus in the Gospel of Matthew, 10:16. We will return to this again in chapter 3.

The Importance of Mystery and Surprise

Self-awareness, as discussed above, is a matter of protection, a positive attribute even though it sounds negative. A more obviously positive reason for developing self-awareness, however, is that it prepares us to expect the unexpected. In the words of Psalm 139, we are both fearfully and wonderfully made. We are a mystery. Although we can never fully understand ourselves, there is much that we can discover and learn if we are willing to fashion for ourselves a discipline of exploring the self. This is not done purely for narcissistic reasons, although as sinners we are certainly prone to have an exaggerated fascination with ourselves. The positive dimension lies in what we can learn about the art of caring for others by focusing regularly and responsibly on learning about ourselves.

Underneath the exterior of every human being there are hidden hurts, distorted motives, and compensating behaviors. There are also unsung joys, unarticulated expressions of gratitude, and wistful hopes that wait hesitantly and expectantly, yearning for expression. As we encounter those dimensions within ourselves, we become more attuned to the needs and fears about power and importance that lurk within the self. To the degree that we are open to learning new things about ourselves, we will be open to and less surprised by the sources of pain and hope within those who come to us in search of some kind of resolution and healing. Though their pains will not be the same as our own, we will find commonality in the struggle. That sense of community paves the way toward healing.

Be aware that mystery here refers not only to the *existence* of this wide array of hurts and hopes. Even more mysterious are the *origins* of those passions. Why do I cry unexpectedly in a movie? Perhaps there are clues from my past that provide partial insight, but it still will be at least a partial mystery to me. What gets in the way of communicating effectively and healthily with those I love? With all I have learned in my chosen field of expertise, that should be easy, shouldn't it? Yet, there are times when I respond with sarcasm or inappropriate nervous laughter, and I will never fully understand where that comes from. It is a mystery. But to the degree that I accept myself as a mystery, I will be less surprised and more accepting when those moments come again. With self-awareness, good intentions, and a bit of luck, I will also be less surprised and more accepting when those outbursts come from others whom I care about and love. Most important of all, I can be grateful that I and we *are* understood in those moments by the God of mystery who created us.

People in the caring professions who become dulled and mechanical in their dealing with others may well have lost touch with, or refuse to look more deeply within, themselves. The cultivation of disciplined self-exploration and awareness keeps us open to new avenues and unexpected discoveries in our work with others. We can rejoice with, hurt with, and continue with these people, but we should not be surprised when something unexpected emerges.

Perhaps the bottom line of this discussion of self-awareness in relationship to mystery is this: To the degree that we are open to further revelation about ourselves and others, we can hope and remain open to surprises and healing.

Summary

Two main purposes shaped this chapter. The first was to invite you into a relatively brief exploration of self without prejudicing you in advance about what you would find. The second was to provide a rationale for the importance of self-awareness in the work of pastoral care in general and in working with sexual issues in particular. Pastoral care of others requires a strong and conscious sense of identity. The discovery of painful sexual issues often requires professional help for ourselves before we can responsibly care for others.

The absence of a clear "sense of self" in professional care-givers can result in great harm to others. In our own day, some of the most profoundly visible hurts are in the sexual arena, in large part because sexuality has to do with both gender issues and intimacy. We will explore these issues further in chapter 2.

For Further Reading

Of course, there are seemingly unlimited resources to be found on identity, intimacy, and exploring the self. Noted below are a few that help focus the suggestions I have already made in this chapter.

For understanding and experiencing the importance of knowing the self in caring for others, I suggest Milton Mayeroff's *On Caring* (New York: Harper & Row, 1971). Almost poetic in its form, it serves as a kind of credo for the caring enterprise.

A book that invites further the self-exploration encouraged here is Anthony Storr's *Solitude: A Return to the Self* (New York: The Free Press, 1988). Storr not only amplifies on the importance of regular time for reflection on the self, but he also suggests a variety of perspectives on the discipline of accomplishing it. Also of encouraging help is *Telling Secrets*, by Frederick Buechner (San Francisco: HarperSanFrancisco, 1991).

Of additional help in working with the relationship between self-knowledge and intimacy is the book mentioned in this chapter by father and son psychiatrists Thomas Patrick Malone and Patrick Thomas Malone, *The Art of Intimacy* (Englewood Cliffs, N.J.: Prentice-Hall, 1987).

If you wish to pursue the exploration of family influences on sexual issues, develop the resource of genograms by reading either *Genograms: The New Tool for Exploring the Personality, Career, and Love Patterns You Inherit* by Emily Marlin (Chicago: Contemporary Books, 1989) or *Genograms in Family Assessment* by M. McGoldrick and R. Gerson (New York: W. W. Norton & Co., 1985). Orientation in focusing more specifically on sexual issues in doing

a genogram can be found in chapter 3, "The Sexual Genogram—
Assessing Family-of-Origin Factors in the Treatment of Sexual
Dysfunction" by Berman and Hof in *Integrating Sex and Marital
Therapy: A Clinical Guide* by Gerald R. Weeks and Larry Hof (New
York: Brunner/Mazel, 1987).

Several other resources are listed below:

Barnhouse, Ruth Tiffany. *Clergy and the Sexual Revolution.*
Washington, D.C.: Alban Institute Publications, 1987.
————. *Identity.* Philadelphia: Westminster Press, 1984.
Dittes, James E. *The Male Predicament: On Being a Man Today.*
San Francisco: Harper & Row, 1985.
Scanzoni, Letha. *Sexuality.* Philadelphia: Westminster Press, 1984.
Schur, Edwin M. *The Awareness Trap: Self-Absorption Instead of
Social Change.* New York: Quadrangle/New York Times,
1976.
Ulanov, Ann Belford. *Receiving Woman: Studies in the Psychology
and Theology of the Feminine.* Philadelphia: Westminster Press,
1981.

2
Gender and Self

In chapter 1 you were invited to do some exploration of your sense of self. That brief journey had a sexual focus. Although not stated specifically in those explorations, you were also exploring what it was and is like to be a man or a woman. Gender is a major shaping force on our sense of self. Gender and self are not the same thing, although it is difficult to separate and define them. The two are intimately and intricately related. In this chapter we will examine some of the connections between one's experience of self as a sexual being and the effect of that experience on the ways we work with and relate to others.

Shaped by our own internal genetic "signals" and by the imposed expectations of others, our perceptions of our gender shape many of the ways in which we act, believe, and feel from early infancy. Our pastoral perspectives and actions will in turn be affected by these influences. Therefore, in continuing our emphasis on self-awareness as an essential component of pastoral care, we will examine these perceptions and other factors from several perspectives.

Psychological Factors Affecting Identity and Lifestyle

Many textbooks in psychology cite a well-known experiment that involved placing an infant in a stroller or playpen in a public place. On some days the child was dressed in pink; on others the same child was dressed in blue. On the days the child was dressed in pink, with few exceptions, the interaction and comments of strangers were soft and tender. Voices were pitched higher, and comments were made about "her" physical characteristics (so soft, so cute, so feminine-looking). These expressions grew out of the perception, based on the pink color of the clothing, that the baby was female. On the days the child was dressed in blue, there were rougher pats on the back, lower-voiced comments, encouraging words about being a good ballplayer (tough little guy, rascal). After all, if clothed in blue, the baby was perceived to be male—and thus was responded to differently!

Of course, any child would be affected by those "cues" from other people. Most of us have formed at least a partial understanding of who we are from such responses. If you went through the exercises in chapter 1, you can probably recall some of those influences that you still carry with you. Those expectations become self-images with which some of us cooperate and against which we may also contend. Gender definitions provide elaborate gradations and norms for intellectual pursuits, choices of work, acceptable activities, and expressions of feelings such as affection and anger. Family rituals and communication patterns often reveal even more specific and differing prescriptions for the behavior of males and females within that family's tradition.

Few would dispute that gender expectations are important factors in conditioning us to behave in particular ways. They are taught to (or imposed on) us early in life, when we are highly impressionable. For many people the resulting patterns of behavior and values attributed to the self become automatic and remain unexamined for many years, if not forever.

Not only does our gender play a significant role in the ways we act, it also affects our conscious beliefs about identity and behavior—indeed, about ourselves. Our unconscious and automatic actions are affected as well. Seldom do we examine those gender expectations that affect our seemingly trivial behavior. When pressed, however, we find that we have also developed deep beliefs and prejudices about gender and sexuality. Certainly, every culture has a variety of conclusions that are drawn about what "man's work" is and what "woman's work" is. The rigidity of those lines varies and, at least in theory, is breaking down in Western cultures, but it is still there. Sometimes the confusion and anxiety of a transitional period, such as we are in now, contribute to intense and rigid demands as people struggle to bring about change or maintain conformity. Members of congregations who are usually open-minded can suddenly find themselves as conflicted over "new" inclusive language in a hymnbook as they are about a denominational position paper on homosexuality. Pastors become quickly involved at such points, because all sides will appeal to religious authority to support their point of view—one more reason that clergy need to be careful and intentional about working on these issues in advance, so that they can work more responsibly with their parishioners.

Both women and men know that if they cross certain cultural or familial boundaries with regard to gender roles, they should be prepared to tolerate more pressure, if not downright discrimination. A good example is the relatively recent history surrounding the ordination of women into the clergy. Until recently, of course, the vast majority of clergy were men. Few mainline denominations had ordained clergywomen prior to the 1950s in the United States. That situation has changed drastically in a relatively short period of time, but not without a great deal of pain and struggle—and it is not over. In fact, now that some of the bigger changes have taken place, the subtle expressions of discrimination are more intense.

Women first gained the right to matriculate in seminary degree programs, then later had to fight for eligibility for ordination. Once that was accomplished, few churches would extend a call to women pastors. Now, many statistics indicate that women can usually get a first call, but all too often they remain in that first pastorate, unable to "move up" or even "move on."

Theological seminaries have had to wrestle with both practical and curricular issues surrounding the changing status of women in the culture and the presence of both genders in the student body. Although women make up from one-third to one-half of most seminary student bodies, the struggle still goes on to gain adequate representation of females on seminary faculties.

In the face of the clear demonstration of women's skills and abilities in ministry, all sorts of unexamined "beliefs" have emerged that interfere with their receiving calls. Examples include: "We can't get a woman in this position on the faculty, because there just aren't any trained women in this field." "How can we call a woman as our minister? Women can't make emergency pastoral calls late at night." "Having a woman in the pulpit might trigger sexual thoughts with men in the congregation." "Married women can't go into ministry, because their husbands couldn't just quit their jobs to follow them somewhere."

While some of these statements may seem ridiculous to us in the 1990s, we are not that far away from the time in which they were effective deterrents to the calling of women into ministry. Indeed, such beliefs are still held in many quarters. Note in all of them that not only are assumptions being made about what is appropriate for women; there are unspoken assumptions also being made about men. Are men "more safe" making calls late at night in a situation of domestic conflict or in a rough neighborhood? Are there plenty of "qualified" men around? Whether you are tempted to laugh, cry, or get angry in the face of all this, the reality is that all of us live with beliefs that are shaped by perceptions about gender.

These beliefs about what we can and cannot do extend beyond vocational choices. We also are shaped in terms of what we believe to be acceptable in informal, social settings. Is it appropriate for a married woman to go out to lunch with a man? The question may seem strange in this day, but it was not in the relatively recent past. And there still are complications. We know from cases involving clergy sexual impropriety that many ministers (mostly men, according to the research) have taken advantage of this "social approval" of their being seen in public places with parishioners of the other gender.

To what degree do we perceive that, as a woman or as a man, we can take the initiative in pursuing a romantic relationship?

Where are the comfort levels stretched when a man or a woman has control of major sums of money? Are lesbian relationships between women somehow more acceptable than gay relationships between men? When pregnancy occurs, either within or outside of marriage, what is the appropriate level of participation and responsibility by the woman and by the man with regard to decisions about abortion, adoption, or keeping the child? All of these things are shaped, in large part, by perceptions connected to gender *and* to culturally assigned prerogatives. Those perceptions then affect our own feelings about ourselves as we "fit in" or refuse to accept those prescriptions. They are intensely present, whether we are aware of it or not, when we as clergy talk with people about making decisions in tough situations.

Biological Factors Affecting Identity and Lifestyle

The situation described above is probably familiar to many readers. In very recent years, however, new information has emerged in the "nature versus nurture" debate, adding to the complexity of sexual issues. As more intricate study has been made of the human brain, fascinating differences are beginning to be identified in its formation and structure in males and females. Some of the findings discussed here are controversial and disturbing—and also exciting and challenging. They add force to the confusing conflict that revolves around sexual roles in our time.

Some scientists are now asserting more emphatically the impact of higher levels of testosterone on the male. Testosterone, they say, is responsible for the "natural," innate aggression of men. As one writer puts it, "We do not teach our boy children to be aggressive—indeed, we vainly try to unteach it" (Moir and Jessel, p. 7). In addition, males, due to the structure of the brain, have greater hand-eye coordination, on average, than females. On the other hand, the average female is able to master finer hand movements. She also responds more sensitively to a wider range of stimuli and thus is often a better judge of character. (It is not just "women's intuition.") Girls learn to speak and read earlier than boys, and they hear better—again because of brain structure.

The differences go on and on, and they are disturbing to some who want to claim that the only differences between men and women have to do with anatomy, not behavior and ability. But the brain is part of the anatomy, and the biological structure of the brain, determined before birth, has characteristics shaped by gender. Consequently, throughout life the brain continues to influence in varying degrees a wide variety of *behavioral* differences between males and females. Those differences, as well as the psychological ones, result in differing experiences of self.

At the time of this writing, a new study emerged that links male homosexual orientation to brain structure, shaped by chemical influences prior to birth. If the findings of this study are confirmed, then the matter of homosexuality will have to be examined anew within the church. Traditional attacks on homosexuality have been based on the assumption that such an orientation is a matter of choice. If the argument holds that homosexual orientation is a choice, then traditional attacks on homosexuality can continue to maintain that through willpower and/or good therapy a heterosexual or celibate choice can and should be made. However, if homosexual orientation is not a matter of choice, then such a religious demand for change would be unfeasible and inhumane.

Most pastors will agree that a frequent phenomenon in their offices is that of a wife complaining about her husband's lack of sensitivity. "He doesn't share his feelings with me," says the wife. "I don't understand what she's talking about," replies the husband. Different definitions of sensitivity are advanced from their respective points of view. So, too, are differences over money management, romance, and child rearing. On and on goes the encounter, with both people protesting that they are misunderstood.

If these biological studies are correct, it is true that men have greater difficulty articulating feelings because of fewer neural connections between the emotional and verbal centers in the brain. If true, is this an excuse for men to withdraw emotionally? Should women give up?

An alert reader will already have said, "Aha. But there are sensitive men and insensitive women. How do the researchers explain that?" The answer is that varying biochemical actions in the womb can result in a variety of "genders" in brains. Less testosterone at a critical period in fetal development can result in a person who has a "female-like" brain, even though the anatomical structure, including genital functioning, is clearly male. The interested reader who wishes to pursue these matters further will find bibliographical references at the end of this chapter.

My point in this section is that sexual, or gender, issues cannot be neatly and cleanly defined. There are a variety of factors, including biological ones, that seem to affect our actions, our choices, our perceptions, and our hopes and dreams. All this must be considered when someone comes to us struggling with actions and feelings that go against what they *believe* ought to be true for them as a man or a woman as they sort out their relationships, their careers, and their lives.

Getting to the Core

Not only are we creatures who *do* and *believe*. We are also creatures who *feel*. Our abilities and beliefs profoundly influence our feelings about self. Psychologically, the terms used to refer to these feelings are "self-regard," "self-esteem," or "self-worth." Here lurks the context for some of the most powerful issues involved in dealing with sexuality. Feelings about the self certainly shape us and what we do. What we feel and how we are able to articulate those feelings have both psychological and biological roots.

Both psychologically and theologically, feelings about the self have to do with our being "true to ourselves," doing what is "fitting," what is *integral* to who we are. Note the interrelatedness of actions, beliefs, and feelings here. That is why the word "integrity" is at the core of a sense of self. It has to do with being able to pull all these factors together into some sort of cohesive whole and live a life that is "self-consistent." An older and fascinating but neglected book on this subject is *Self-Consistency* by Prescott Lecky (1961). The theological term would be "faithful." Is my feeling about myself one that carries a sense of integrity, of having been faithful to who I am? If not, then I am likely to be plagued with feelings of worthlessness, guilt, and shame. Women often suffer negative feelings about self because of prohibitions or denigrations that are placed on them culturally and psychologically. Men often suffer negative feelings because of their inability effectively to articulate and work with what is taking place at the emotional level. Again, many of these people find their way to a pastor's study to struggle with "bad feelings about myself" or a marriage. Perhaps they have found a lifestyle that seems "right," but they are plagued by feelings of it being "not right." There is something that still comes through, spoken or unspoken, in people when feelings about the self are bad. Many of them want to turn for reassurance to a religious frame of reference.

Sadly enough, "negative" feelings, when expressed, are not always in proportion to what is going on. The exaggerated values and expectations that have shaped us lead to equally exaggerated feelings in response. Thus, our problems are compounded.

A medical doctor was overcome by his inability to relieve the emotional pain of a young friend whose mother had died. It was not that he was hurting *for* the young man. Rather, he thought that it was his own duty "as a man" and as a mentor to know how to keep his junior colleague from hurting so much. It soon became clear that it was a *sexual* issue for him—not in the narrow sense in which we normally use the word. He saw himself as not wise enough, not strong enough, not *manly* enough, to do what needed to be done. If he were a "real man," he thought, he could "fix it."

It is in these moments of disparity between what "is" and what "ought to be" that persons often seek help or clarification about what is going on. Sometimes, because their pain has become visible and cannot be ignored, clergy take the initiative and invite them to "come over and talk about it." There are other times when pastors are surprised at being approached by the person who looks "so well put together." The pain was well concealed until it was "confessed" in the privacy of the pastoral relationship.

Certainly, feelings about the self are not solely determined by gender issues, but some of the most powerful feelings about the self are. A young seminarian sat in a pastor's office and described his decision to go into the ministry. With tears running down his face, he detailed time after time in his life when he had been poor in sports, had avoided fights and been teased for it, had been embarrassed at weeping in front of other males or frightened when in the face of danger. Like the physician described above, he said, "I'm just not *manly*, so I decided to become a minister." Look at the feelings about self that were triggered by actions and feelings that seemed out of accord with what seemed to be "maleness" (not to mention the feelings about the vocation of ministry itself and the feelings that may have been generated in the pastor who was listening). Look at the perception of himself that is carried into ministry—a forced option because of his perceived failure as a man. Little integrity could be experienced in living out such a choice.

Or, take the situation of a never-married, responsible, and very meticulous forty-two-year-old woman who came to her pastor's office by appointment. She spoke of the increasing frequency of her being awakened over the last six months by dreams of being smothered. Over a period of time the dream became clearer. A face, hovering over her, had become more and more visible. It was her father's. With horror she realized that the two of them had had an incestuous relationship, now long repressed. She was not a partner in it—she was the victim. Nonetheless, a shy, guilt-laden lifestyle had grown from that forgotten experience. One result had been avoidance of relationships because she did not feel worthy as a woman, but until now she had not known why. Since realizing this part of her history, she was further bewildered by the strong feeling that she was permanently "tainted." She had not been able to acknowledge it or talk about it until the new female pastor at her church befriended her.

Those feelings about self were deeply embedded by the sexual experience. They were compounded by another perception that she had gained from her mother—that it must have been her fault for somehow "tempting" her father, because that is what women "do." All the previous shaping from the complex mixture of gender issues that we have discussed was finally exposed. Then the healing could begin.

A Theological Digression: Finitude and Sin

At this point a theological digression seems appropriate as we take up the task of bringing theology, psychology, and our biology and body chemistry into interplay with each other. In the examples given above, the individuals were to some degree helpless. The first young man did not *choose* to be sensitive and deeply affected by pain and conflict. Nor did the second choose to be a poor athlete. In like manner, the woman did not invite her father to molest her sexually, nor could she have had the physical strength to prevent it. But all three of these people felt somehow ashamed and responsible for what happened.

While some might say that these people did have some potential control, I maintain that overall they were not fully in control of what they felt and what they did. They were relatively powerless, at least in the face of biological predisposition and strong social definitions of what it is to be a man and what it is to be a woman. The man is to be tough, athletic, and thick skinned. The woman is to be gentle, pure, and weak, yet she is to remain "unviolated." Failure by either men or women to "measure up" to these cultural norms generates deep feelings of guilt and shame.

When these sex role stereotypes are not upheld, for whatever reason, a frequent result is deep and abiding injury to the self. After all, the self has "bought in" at some level. Thus, all of these people are left with a feeling of "culpability," as if they did have power.

Here the crucial theological separation between finitude and sin becomes very important. Unfortunately, it is a distinction too often lost, compounding the powerful feelings described in the examples.

As human beings, we are finite. We are limited creatures. Created in the image of God, we are reflections of God. But as images, we are, by definition and by creation, *not* infinite. We are not all-powerful. Things happen to us that we cannot control. Our nature, our personalities—each has expressions and characteristics over which we have limited power. We cannot fully change ourselves in the ways we would like. As noted earlier, biological evidence continues to emerge that partially confirms this.

On the basis of all these factors, biological, psychological, and theological, I believe that within limits the seminarian *cannot help* those characteristics that he described. But, he treats them as if he were guilty of having made bad choices and thus labels himself a failure. The woman *could not help* being molested by her father. Yet, she treats the event as if she could have prevented it. Both persons respond to their limits, their finitude, as if they were sinful. But we are not *guilty* for being limited. That is simply a "given" about who we are as human beings. But when finitude is treated emotionally as if it is sin, then linked with the deep roots of sexuality, significant emotional intensity goes chaotically surging through the self.

A full-blown doctrine of sin is beyond the scope of our task here. There are many dimensions and expressions of sin, including such factors as the idolatry of self, the demand that others be like oneself, and the refusal to value differences. Our concern here is the perception and experience of sin that govern these people's feelings about themselves. The most common understanding of sin *in daily life* probably revolves around a sense of "doing wrong." There is an element of perceived *choice*, thus an assumption that control was, or is, possible. Because of the misperception that control was available, physician, seminarian, and abused woman live with a sense of shame and guilt for circumstances largely beyond their control. And, they are left with a perception and experience of themselves as unworthy, bad people—sinful. Their sense of self—their identity—is thereby distorted as they wrestle with some form of self-recrimination for having failed.

The refusal or inability to distinguish between finitude and sin, between helplessness and choice, results in much of the pain and suffering that people experience. That is particularly true in the already emotionally charged sphere of sexuality. The inability to make this distinction is in itself a testimony to human finitude. We know, for instance, that people under intense stress or anxiety, in the absence of self-awareness, begin to lose the ability to make distinctions. A focused sense of self is lost. Choices and perceptions blur, and the ability to see alternatives fades. The power of sexuality, its depth of feeling, often makes it difficult to separate feeling from fact, rationality from emotionality. Discernment fades in the face of such overwhelming force.

We must be careful in our discussion of sin and finitude to avoid the temptation to pronounce people always as helpless victims in matters of feelings and sexual choices. There are people who are abused in spite of their best efforts to avoid it. It is also true that there are people who claim abuse because they know it can be used to their advantage. While there are cases in which the distinction between finitude and sin will be clearly visible, there probably are far more situations in which it is not possible to separate them clearly. The point here is that our all-too-human temptation is to put things in terms of either-or. Yet, to do so is to place people under horrible burdens of pain and self-recrimination. If everything that happens to me is interpreted as my responsibility, thus my fault, then superhuman expectations have been placed on me. We human beings are just not that strong!

We *need* help from outside of ourselves. There is relief, otherwise known as grace, in knowing we cannot do everything or take responsibility for everything. Here lies the context for admission of our finitude, for testimony to our need for community, for acknowledgment of our need for God's grace and power, and our need for pastoral care. In sexual matters, in particular, we need to look at ourselves with the knowledge that, while guilty in some areas, there are other experiences that are simply beyond our control. The appropriate response then is not guilt, but grief. Far too often persons are condemned instead of comforted. They live a life characterized by guilt or shame instead of feeling accepted as they mourn losses over which they had no control.

When seen and experienced, the difference between finitude and sin does not give license to "do what we feel because we can't help it, anyway." Rather, there emerges a sense of freedom to look at ourselves more clearly and to focus ourselves on the growth that is possible and redemptive in our lives, rather than being chained to old wounds that dictate a life of emotional imprisonment.

The Way We Relate to Others

You are seeing, I hope, a progression of thought as we explore the ways in which sexuality shapes our sense of self. Our actions are influenced from birth by biological, psychological, cultural, and familial issues and perceptions related to our sexual gender. Our current experiences of acting and being acted upon by others further shapes feelings about self. The feelings we hold about self shape the ways we relate to others.

If a person's perception of self is reasonably healthy and intact, there will be relative comfort in connecting with others in ways that are authentic and reasonably confident. If not, she or he will develop a variety of techniques, defenses, and facades to hide the sense of self that is such a source of shame. In extreme cases, people feel fragile enough to find ways to seal themselves off from relationships altogether.

While gender perceptions affect our involvement with others in a general way, there are more specific dynamics that arise when sexual (not necessarily genital) involvement occurs. If one's self is perceived to be of little worth, then one is even more prone to "use" his or her body to gain attention and regard. Overestimation or underestimation of self can lead to "teasing" others sexually in an effort to control them. Such control of others serves to avoid intimacy with them. The manipulative power of sexuality can be used to keep relationships in a dominant-subservient style, rather than in mutuality and partnership. In other words, sex is used to get the desired job, the desired status, the desired power—in a sometimes desperate quest for self-assurance. The quest, however, is self-defeating, because in the very act of seeking control, the person is cut off from what is needed most—a caring and trusting partnership with another or others. And, of course, in the attempt to be fully in control, the person is even cutting the self off from intimacy with God.

The number of ways in which relationships are affected by sexuality is many and varied, and the range is from beautiful peaks of intimacy to vulgar degradation and hurt. Sexuality can enhance and deepen relationships or be used to avoid and hurt.

The Bible frequently portrays the rich expressiveness possible between two lovers:

> Arise, my love, my fair one, and come away;
> for now the winter is past,
>   the rain is over and gone.
> The flowers appear on the earth;
>   the time of singing has come,
> and the voice of the turtledove is heard in our land.
>   —*Song of Solomon 2:10b–12*

Rollo May, on the other hand, speaks of the pain experienced by others dealing with sexuality: "Few patients seem repressed. In fact, they have many sexual partners. . . . what our patients do complain of is lack of feeling and passion. . . . So much sex and so little meaning or even fun in it!" (*Love and Will*, p. 40).

To Be a Sexual Self Is to Be Different

Part of the power involved in understanding sexuality and self lies in the fact that our sexual identity is largely a matter of differences. When we think of those differences, we are first aware of the dissimilarities between male and female. We become conscious of being a self by recognizing our separateness or differentness from others. Those differences serve several functions. They lead to self-realization and open doors to intrigue and fascination with both our own self and the self that is different from us.

THE PASTOR'S RESPONSIBILITY FOR SELF-AWARENESS

At the same time, in our desire to avoid isolation, we look for similarities, points of commonality. Very soon then, identifications are formed with same-sexed people and the nature of differentness from other-sexed people is further clarified. The most obvious differences and similarities have to do with visible factors, namely our bodies. So, as a self, each of us learns what is different about us with regard to some people and what in us is like some other people. Identity, or a sense of self, evolves partly from experiences of similarity and dissimilarity. In recognition of people like ourselves, we begin to develop a sense of association and community. From that association, awareness dawns about how "we" are akin, over against "them." A problem develops at this point if identity development halts and begins to hinge on having to maintain a sense of "over against-ness" in order to feel good about oneself. I prefer to speak of the "other" sex, rather than the "opposite" sex. At least symbolically, it moves away from viewing the two as having to be "in opposition to" each other.

The development of a sense of self involves subtleties beyond physical bodies. Otherness can be and is found among people of the same gender. In God's design, differences are an exceptionally important feature. Not only is there wide variety among us human beings; there is also a vast assortment in geography, plant life, animal life, and microscopic existence. Differences confront us with our uniqueness and importance, and at the same time with mystery and lack of control. And so we both celebrate and tremble at the same time. Again, in the words of the Psalmist, we are both "fearfully and wonderfully made" (Psalm 139:14).

That capacity to experience opposing feelings and reactions (fear and wonder) toward the same object at the same time is another characteristic that both enriches our emotional life and makes us uneasy. We can in the same moment love and be angry at a friend, a lover, a child, a parent. Differences are within us as well as around us, and they are difficult to organize and understand.

In the face of these differences we are prone to try to take control or to manufacture harmony. Attempts may be made to demand sameness in belief, preference, or even dress! It is an attempt to reduce our life experiences to a "manageable" or "managed" level. That is abundantly true with regard to our sexuality. Those very differences that offer the potential for ecstasy, enrichment, and/or enjoyment also create the context for anxiety, fear, and anger. The path over which our developing sense of self has traveled greatly affects our ability to enjoy and respect the differences or to view the differences as threatening.

If our sense of worth has become dependent on agreement or sameness with others, then our relationships will be constant struggles for control or seduction in a false quest for peace. If our sense of worth builds to an appreciation of differences and willingness to learn through exploration and discovery, then our relationships can become welcome opportunities for growth.

Differences, as noted earlier, are real and appear in many ways. One recent book illustrates the matter well. In her book *You Just Don't Understand*, Deborah Tannen confirms issues that have been identified by other writers. Men in conversation are more likely to talk asymmetrically, seeking status, enjoying competition, attempting solutions. Women are more likely to speak symmetrically, seeking community, enjoying mutuality, sharing feelings. Without accepting or at least acknowledging those differences, much misunderstanding takes place between men and women. Assumptions are made about the motives, purpose, sensitivity, and ability of the other. A genuine cultural gap exists. When not understood or at least appreciated and accepted, such a gap breeds hurt and conflict.

If such misunderstanding takes place in conversation, consider what takes place in more intimate encounters—not only genital ones but also in the sharing of more vulnerable concerns. These differences emphasize again the observations described above. Our actions, beliefs, and feelings are all shaped by our understanding of who we are *and* by our perception of the genuine differences between the genders and between selves. The "otherness" becomes both a source for growth and a repository for pain. Our hope in pastoral care is that the balance can tip toward the growth side.

The reader may rightly wonder at this point if we are really talking about sexuality in all this. The answer is "yes." While there are certainly more differences than sexual ones, most other differences are conditioned further by our experiences and interpretations of maleness and femaleness. And this is to speak only of the more routine activities of our lives. When differences are amplified even more by specific experiences such as rape, incest, homosexuality, and teenage pregnancy, the potential for pain and misunderstanding grows immensely.

Differences bring, if not drive, people to pastors. They come because they are seeking reconciliation—a very theological and pastoral word. They come also because the differences that separate them are, in many ways, mysterious to them. The mystery casts a religious shadow over the issue. Feeling out of control and misunderstood, they come seeking reconciliation with others and within the self. It is no wonder that pastors need to be aware of the variables that may be at work in the pain and confusion.

Our Bodies and Our Selves

A number of years ago a book was published by the Boston Women's Health Collective titled *Our Bodies, Ourselves* (New York: Simon & Schuster, 1973). A revised edition has been published more recently (*The New Our Bodies, Ourselves*, 1985). Though not theological in its concern, the title is absolutely appropriate for a theological discussion. We cannot know ourselves apart from knowing our bodies. We are incarnated creatures, and our spirit cannot be separated from this earthly frame. It is through our bodies that we see, hear, taste, smell, and touch all that is around us. Those cues influence our understanding of ourselves, the world, other people, and our place in relationship to them. Erik Erikson, in discussing the concept of identity, once wrote that the task of identity formation revolves around our bringing our own perception of ourselves and the perceptions of others about us into some sort of congruity. That includes our perceptions of our bodies. James Nelson, in his helpful book *Embodiment*, refers to human beings as "body-selves." These writers make more graphic the reality that our bodies make up a great deal of and are inseparable from our self-definition. Certainly we are more than flesh, but our bodies extend, receive, respond, and generate much of what we know and believe about ourselves. How do we feel about our bodies? What is the internal response to praise of our bodies? What is the response to criticism? We use our bodies to explore relationships, to "check out" and to give signals about the kind of relationship we want and do not want with others.

Think again about some of the observations you made in going through the exercises in chapter 1. Look at the immense variety of signals communicated through body language. Think of those people you touch and those you do not touch. A handshake is the formal expression in many cultures of regard and friendliness, or at least the agreement and assurance that we will not (or cannot, while shaking hands) knife each other in the back. A shake of the hand accompanied by a grip of the arm by the other hand takes it one step further. Next might come an embrace or a kiss. The length and kind of embrace or kiss gives further confirmation, or sets limits, about the level of caring and intimacy. There are a variety of subtle but clear signals for which we look in eye contact or body language as we seek to understand the regard in which we are held or as we seek to communicate to the other person the regard in which we hold them. We also know the capability that bodily expressions have to hurt someone. Care should be exercised because of the meanings associated with touch. It is possible to tease persons, to be flirtatious, to take advantage of their vulnerability. A touch can conjure up fantasies and hope for more of a relationship than is willingly being offered. If such behavior is done frivolously or for self-aggrandizement, then the other has been treated in a dehumanizing way—a way that defaces the image of God in that person.

All Things Working Together

Paul, in his letter to the Romans, says, "We know that all things work together for good for those who love God, who are called according to his purpose" (Rom. 8:28). As sexual beings, we are composed of a complex variety of members that are designed to work together: feelings, beliefs, actions; body, mind, and spirit. When these dimensions of our identity work together with a sense of purpose, then we experience something of the richness for which God intended us. When there is a sense of "having it all together," a man or a woman can look at the world with appreciation and joy.

When these dimensions of identity are divided, assaulted, and/or abused, the pain is excruciating. A man or a woman remains on guard and rigid in the face of an ever-perceived threat of attack. Freedom and joy are lost in the midst of manipulation. A sense of worth collapses in the face of expectations for perfection. The parts of the self are used, rather than enjoyed; constantly evaluated rather than trusted; burned out instead of being given time to rest.

Human life is full of experiences and forces that push and pull us in our search for identity. Because of the particular, often frightening, power that surrounds sexual identity, too much is unspoken, denied, avoided. When the pain becomes too much, people are prone to react in exaggerated ways, increasing the pain out of a misguided and desperate attempt to avoid it. Hence, the importance of educated, committed, self-aware persons to render pastoral care.

The first part of this book has set a stage for the importance of working with sexual issues. As I said earlier, in spite of the public furor or the public silence, still there are people searching for a private and safe place to seek understanding, a sanctuary. In that place, often a pastoral relationship, they need to sort out things that they have ignored or fought for too long. When that can be done, the relationship becomes a "sacred place," where all things are speakable. Intimacy, spirituality, boundaries, integrity, communication, sense of self—all can be spoken in the belief that in the vulnerability of speaking, their voice will be heard. The person who listens should be someone who understands the intensity, recognizes the complexity, and knows that there are no easy answers to this pilgrimage that we call life. Such a person must also be self-aware enough to sense when it is important to listen and recognize the right moment to speak. Such wisdom is not as rare as you might think, but the development of that wisdom takes discipline. I hope I have encouraged the wisdom in a general way in these first two chapters. While I will offer information and suggestions for particular issues and situations in part 2, one more chapter seems necessary to look specifically at matters of pastoral conduct.

Suggestions for Further Reading

A variety of books are helpful in looking at the issues of masculinity and femininity. One that summarizes well the research into brain structure is Anne Moir and David Jessel's *Brain Sex: The Real Difference between Men and Women* (New York: Lyle Stuart, 1991). A second that deals with masculine and feminine differences from the perspective of communication is Deborah Tannen's best-selling *You Just Don't Understand: Women and Men in Conversation* (New York: William Morrow & Co., 1990).

Some psychological works written some time ago that deal with identity helpfully though without specific attention to gender issues include Prescott Lecky's *Self-Consistency: A Theory of Personality* (Seattle: The Shoe String Press, 1961), and Andras Angyal's *Neurosis and Treatment: A Holistic Theory* (New York: John Wiley & Sons, 1965). Erik Erikson's *Identity and the Life Cycle: Selected Papers* (New York: International Universities Press, 1959) is a classic work on identity. It must be balanced by work that takes women's gender issues into account, such as Carol Gilligan's *In a Different Voice: Psychological Theory and Women's Development* (Cambridge: Harvard University Press, 1982). Helpful connections between the body and the sense of self are provided by the book mentioned earlier, *The New Our Bodies, Ourselves,* by the Boston Women's Health Collective (New York:

Simon & Schuster, 1985). A number of helpful chapters on identity issues and family-of-origin influences can be found in the more recent *The Changing Family Life Cycle: A Framework for Family Therapy*, edited by Betty Carter and Monica McGoldrick (Needham Heights, Mass.: Allyn and Bacon, 1989). Helpful explorations from a number of different systems perspectives are to be found in *Handbook of Family Therapy*, volumes 1 and 2, edited by Alan S. Gurman and David P. Kniskern (New York: Brunner/Mazel, 1991). See also Rollo May, *Love and Will* (New York: W. W. Norton & Co., 1969).

Pastoral and theological treatments are numerous. Several of the more helpful ones include:

Borrowdale, Anne. *Distorted Images: Misunderstandings between Men and Women*. Louisville, Ky.: Westminster/John Knox Press, 1991.

Browne, Peter. *The Body and Society: Men, Women and Sexual Renunciation in Early Christianity*. New York: Columbia University Press, 1988.

Cahill, Lisa Sowle. *Between the Sexes: Foundations for a Christian Ethics of Sexuality*. Philadelphia: Fortress Press, 1985.

Countryman, L. William. *Dirt, Greed, and Sex: Sexual Ethics in the New Testament and Their Implications for Today*. Philadelphia: Fortress Press, 1988.

Jewett, Paul King. *Man as Male and Female: A Study in Sexual Relationships from a Theological Point of View*. Grand Rapids: Eerdmans, 1975.

Nelson, James B. *Between Two Gardens: Reflections on Sexuality and Religious Experience*. New York: Pilgrim Press, 1983.

———. *Body Theology*. Louisville, Ky.: Westminster/John Knox Press, 1992.

———. *Embodiment: An Approach to Sexuality and Christian Theology*. Minneapolis: Augsburg Publishing House, 1978.

Phipps, William E. *Genesis and Gender: Biblical Myths of Sexuality and Their Cultural Impact*. New York: Praeger, 1989.

Sanford, John A. *The Invisible Partners: How the Male and Female in Each of Us Affects Our Relationships.* New York: Paulist Press, 1980.

Terrien, Samuel L. *Till the Heart Sings: A Biblical Theology of Manhood and Womanhood.* Philadelphia: Fortress Press, 1985.

3

Climate, Conduct, and Referral

Regardless of the agenda and circumstances that have brought pastor and parishioner together for pastoral care, certain fundamental issues are vital to the well-being of the pastoral relationship. Because these matters are basic to pastoral work, the discussion here is likely to be more of a reminder than new information. Nonetheless, because of the possible discomfort often raised by discussion of sexual issues, the climate, or context, of pastoral care, pastoral conduct, and referral are discussed here as one more dimension of consciousness-raising.

In considering the climate of pastoral care, we need to look again at our own personal situation, then the context in which care is given, and finally the spirit or attitude that informs our approach to those who come seeking aid.

Get Yourself Together

Dealing with issues of sexuality today is among the most agonizing and taxing of the circumstances that pastors face with individuals. The drama and intensity of people's feelings, including your own, make it very difficult to provide the wisdom and discernment that are needed. However, theological perspective certainly reminds us that this intensity should be no surprise. Our gender is deeply embedded within our sense of who we are—a part of God's image—and is vital to our own self-understanding and to our sense of worth and connectedness with others. When people struggle with sexual issues, they are facing the fact of their creatureliness (including their finitude, discussed in the previous chapter) and their sense of worth as a child of God.

That is heavy stuff! So, the first task is to take a deep breath, then pray for the restraint and ability to be "with" people, wherever they may be. Our prayer should include a petition for the strength to avoid launching into a mechanical attempt to "fix" whatever is wrong, because fixing is not the focus. Healing is. Any healing that occurs will take place over a long period of time, and we may be just one small part of it. Moreover, the specific shape and direction of that healing are not likely to be known for a good while.

Having focused and prepared to step into a privileged and painful role as pastor to the people involved, our next task is to use our ability to provide acceptance and maintain calm to foster a similar frame of mind in the parishioner. This calm is sometimes referred to as a "relatively nonanxious presence"—the maintenance of a posture that enables one to step back and reflect on what is happening from a distance without becoming too intensely involved. John Cobb has called this ability to stand outside of the self one of the marks of our transcendence, the ability to muster some, though not total, objectivity about what is going on—another reflection of being created in God's image. To get in touch with that capacity assures troubled parties that some control and choices are possible in spite of seemingly out-of-control circumstances.

Create a Safe and Comfortable Context

The suggestions about managing ourselves aim toward the creation of a psychologically and physically safe place for the party or parties seeking care. Passion and intensity are characteristic when dealing with issues of sexuality. In the face of strong emotion, it is important to invite people into a pastoral climate.

Creating a safe place may sound like an obvious thing to do, but it is not easy. The more difficult the situation, the more complex is the cultivation of a spirit of trust and safety. Several concrete things can be done to foster such an environment.

Time

First, it is important to allow time for the story to be told in the person's own way. If the available time is short, say so. Otherwise, the pastor's edginess and anxiety about the limited time may lead the person, probably already apprehensive, to perceive the uneasiness as discomfort, disapproval, or preferring not to deal with the concern. That is the last thing you want to convey to someone who has probably had to work up tremendous courage to come in the first place.

If time is limited, suggest another meeting, perhaps before engaging in any further conversation. To do so provides assurance of your commitment and interest. Making that next time soon will give further assurance of your willingness and interest.

An hour, more or less, is a good length of time for an appointment. Fatigue and repetitiveness begin to enter after that period. Finally, stick to the length of time originally suggested. People often save some items for the end, because they *do not* want to go into them at length. If the pastor says in response to a new issue, "Well, we can certainly take some more time to talk about *that*," then one of two disquieting things will probably occur. First, the pastor will have unintentionally taught the person how to get the pastor to spend more time with him or her: Bring up something dramatic! That can invite manipulative ploys later. Or the extension of time may "mess up" the person's plan to introduce a topic and then think further before discussing it in depth. While pastors do not spend the majority of their time as professional therapists, it is well to remember there are good reasons for the "therapeutic hour." It provides comfort and safe boundaries for the person who needs to open up at her or his own pace.

Privacy

Be careful about allowing interruptions during a pastoral conversation. Interruptions include telephone calls, knocks on the door, questions relayed in, or the pastor's own eccentricities (such as playing with a pencil or staring out the window for long periods of time). Such things may signal the other person not to communicate in depth or with emotion, because of his or her anxiety over being stopped or ignored in midstream. To allow such interruptions tells the person that undivided attention is not available. Divided attention communicates divided loyalties and lack of dependability or cooperation.

When Questions Are Not Helpful

Early questions may seem too curious to an already anxious person. Questions, in fact, guide the conversation and tell the speaker what the listener considers "interesting" and what the listener does not. Do not prematurely narrow your own vision or that of the person who has come to you. This is no time to unintentionally and hastily close out any perspectives on what is going on or what needs to be faced. A caring person communicates vividly by listening fully before narrowing the focus. The hurting person experiences the seriousness with which he or she is being taken. Once heard fully, and with few interruptions, a person can be led into more focused discussion and exploration of his or her story.

Self-Awareness

A further important aspect of providing a safe and comfortable context has to do with the self-awareness discussed earlier in this book. A "safe harbor" is provided by a calm, inviting, and understanding self who is neither surprised nor offended by what is said. This is not to say a mature pastor will not be troubled by things that are said. Moral and ethical viewpoints are not being set aside permanently. But, to ease the fears of judgment that probably lurk in the imagination of the other person, a willingness to suspend judgment until all is known must be evident. Pouncing on the first distressing item helps no one and tends to curtail a person's story.

So What?

Much described here involves good listening skills. A requirement that I have often wanted to place on seminary students making first pastoral visits in a hospital or parishioner's home is this: Enter into a conversation for ten minutes without asking a question or giving a word of advice. This is suggested here as a way of contributing to the building of a safe and comfortable environment. *Restrain yourself.* There will be time later to sort things through in more detail.

Encourage a Spirit of Moral Inquiry

Several years ago, in his book *The Moral Context of Pastoral Care*, Don Browning effectively introduced the term "moral inquiry" to describe pastoral care when it is being carried out well. More has been written since then by Browning and others, but he was among the first in recent years to declare that pastoral care has settled for too limited a range of skills and responsibilities. Listening was and is important. But when the listening has been genuine, pathways open for more direct and specific exploration.

Let me quickly emphasize, having just cautioned the reader about asking questions, that moral inquiry is not an inquisition. Rather, it is an attitude and an orientation that builds on the spirit of trust developed by sensitive listening. There is an opportunity within this safe context to engage the issues of sexuality from a variety of angles. Please note that the phrase is moral *inquiry*. There is no intention to legislate or prescribe morality. Rather, the aim is to guide a conversation already characterized by listening and trust through an exploration of various points of view and their impact on a particular situation. In this spirit of inquiry and mutual exploration, the pastor can introduce subject matter from any of a number of these "angles of vision."

One angle is to explore the range of knowledge and information the person has about the sexual issues being explored. The variety of perspectives discussed in each of the following chapters can be a source for introducing the person or persons to a wider range of ideas and data to develop deeper understanding and alternate coping strategies.

Persons struggling with sexual issues often find themselves

confused and discouraged about what is going on. Frequently, they are also afraid there is only one acceptable way to view their plight, or there is only one ultimate outcome. Information about other aspects of the issue can bring a sense of relief that there are no certain answers. A newly fostered spirit of exploration becomes an energizing opportunity—a welcome relief from the dread of some immediate pronouncement of sin or grace.

Often people come to the pastor asking him or her to "choose up sides" on an issue. The pastor who falls into that trap relinquishes the opportunity to render deeper and more enduring pastoral care. That in itself is another angle of vision. Not only is information offered, but also along with it comes a different context for processing that information—a place where there is freedom and invitation to explore, rather than pressure to prematurely agree to or settle on something.

Another angle of vision lies in the invitation to people to engage in the same sort of exploration of self that you were encouraged to do in the first chapter. To look at one's own shaping influences, to question, affirm, and seek further clarity, offers fresh perspective. That, too, is a moral inquiry—reflection on our own "roots."

Pastoral Conduct

One current manifestation of sexual confusion (and abuse) is the unfolding awareness of the sexual advantage some professionals take of patients, clients, and parishioners. The clinical term often used in evaluating such actions is "boundaries." If a patient submits to the sexual overtures of a professional counselor, then her or his personal boundaries have been crossed and appropriate physical and emotional distance has not been maintained. The professional, however, is the guilty party for failing to maintain such crucial limits on involvement with a client or parishioner.

Of course, one frequent reason for seeking professional help is the very experience of having been regularly "invaded" because of inability to maintain ego boundaries in the face of "power plays" by others. The inability is itself an expression of collapse in the face of "assault."

What is sad, even angering, is that in such circumstances the professional may also violate personal boundaries and become one more invading enemy doing harm to personhood and integrity. An essential characteristic of the relationship between doctor and patient, counselor and counselee, pastor and parishioner, is that conversations and treatment occur in a "safe place." The safe place is the relationship itself, one in which the professional is aware of and respectful of the patient or parishioner's vulnerability. It is incumbent on the "expert" to maintain his or her own boundaries, thus creating a context within which the counselee can both experience the richness of healthy relationships and begin to develop and maintain her or his own limits. Over time, if growth is successful, there will be less and less need for another person to construct or maintain these boundaries, because the person will be capable of creating and maintaining them independently.

As stated in the first chapter, the professional, if not self-aware, is more subject to the desires and temptations faced by all of us as human beings. Sexual feelings, needs for intimacy, and desire for control often emerge with surprising urgency. If unfamiliar with that mysterious part of the self, the person in a responsible and professional position falls prey to powerful forces and then violates the integrity of the care that he or she is expected to render. Not knowing is not an excuse. Responsible self-awareness is a prerequisite for one who assumes the role of caregiver.

Setting Limits

There have been a number of publications attempting to define codes of conduct for practitioners in their relationships to clients and/or parishioners. Of course, a set of rules does not fully capture the ideal. Responsible relatedness is more a matter of character and the heart than something that can be reduced to rational expression. Nonetheless, the pursuit of codes is one means of attempting to give expression at least to minimal expectations.

This book will not propose a comprehensive code, although references are provided at the end of this chapter for the reader who wishes to see examples of such attempts. The purpose here is to alert the pastor to areas for scrutiny—again, with the emphasis on self-awareness. Regular introspection and conversation with colleagues contribute significantly to the protection of both self and others within the intimacy that is attendant to dealing with sexuality. The rhetoric of boundaries will be used to illustrate the various ways in which a relationship should be both maintained and scrutinized.

Boundaries of Space

Space has to do with place, and the place at which people meet communicates a great deal about the nature of the relationship that they share. An office, for instance, communicates formality and focus. Work is being done there, and the place of work and the kind of work are known publicly. People who are there have come for a purpose, and the purposes are at least generally defined. Those purposes, defined by the space in which they are accomplished, provide definition and boundaries.

When people come to the pastor's study, therefore, the place itself sets certain expectations and guidelines for behavior and subject matter. Those limits provide a sense of safety. That safety then provides freedom to explore sensitive matters with little fear of harm.

A person's home defines a different set of boundaries. On the one hand, it is less in the public eye. Even so, it is a reminder of the relationships that exist within its walls and the expectations and commitments that those relationships represent. Thus, the home may very well be a safe place. On the other hand, the suggestion of an "out-of-the-way" place, such as an intimate restaurant in the evening, communicates its own set of expectations and freedoms. A clergyperson needs to be very sensitive to the messages being conveyed by such a choice of place.

The point here is that a wise pastor uses place judiciously. A place is more than just a geographical area. It is a reminder of relationships, of role definitions, of personal and professional promises made. The place at which a pastor chooses to meet communicates intentions to the other person and can set limits, encourage openness, arouse feelings, or threaten to invade. In the same way, the arrangement of furniture and seating patterns signal levels of distance, safety, or inappropriate closeness. Be sensitive to these nonverbal but very real factors involved in place.

Many female clergy find having lunch with a parishioner is a more private, less formal, time "to talk." If subjects arise that need more in-depth discussion, then a following time can be arranged at the office. Again, there may be a male/female difference here. Some male clergy may feel that "doing lunch" is less desirable than making the rounds on the golf course, for instance. Many a personal and theological discussion has taken place on the fairway.

Boundaries of Time

As does space, time communicates. To give people extra time tells them that they or their situation is special. In that sense, pastors are genuine *givers* of time, unlike other professional people (including pastoral counselors in private practice) who, in effect, sell their time. Pastors, then, are in a relatively unique position in that there is no fee for the care and counsel they offer. Consequently, there is more room to misinterpret what the giving of time means. On the one hand, this is a privilege. There is freedom to "give" time to those who appear to need it most, without regard to their capacity to pay. On the other hand, the giving of time to people may be interpreted by them as an indication of a kind of specialness that the pastor does not have in mind!

Be careful, but not stingy, in the amount of time given to others. If a parishioner discovers that time seems to be given in proportion to the drama of the story, opportunities for some control over the pastor may be seen. An offer to meet at times other than "regular" hours may give rise to the perception that intimacy is the message rather than willingness to be available. Certainly there are occasions on which people are rightly seen early or late. But if a pattern begins to develop, consider what might be read into what is taking place.

Unfortunately, there are no simple rules to be laid out here, except to be careful. If you find yourself giving more and more time, ask yourself why.

Boundaries of Language

Not only are matters of space and time important, but choice of words also carries both opportunity and danger. Educated pastors may be aware of the complexity and technical nature of language but in conversation forget that other people have their own meanings for the vocabulary employed. Use of the word "love" is a case in point. We may assure a person of our love and care only to discover later that our words were heard as a proposal of a more intimate relationship. Assurance to someone that he or she is "special" to us may be interpreted as permission for them to call us and/or show up unannounced wherever we may be.

The literature on active listening reminds us of the importance of getting feedback from people to determine if they (and we) have heard what is intended. Such clarification is important "maintenance" in counseling and caring relationships.

Boundaries of Touch

It would be a rare professional person who is not sensitized today to the ways in which touch can be misused and misunderstood. The "pastoral hug" can be reported later as abusive and inappropriately "familiar." It is a shame that we need to be extra sensitive to matters of touching, but we live in a world in which touch is too often considered invasive instead of supportive. On the other hand, sensitivity to touch is a reminder of what a powerful and healing force it can be when offered with care.

It is important to be careful about whom we touch and how or where we touch them. A pat on the hand may be preferable to a hug until we know the person better and have more comprehension of her or his response to these exchanges that take place through touch. Remember that interpretations of touch vary not only with personal preference but with cultural norms as well.

Boundaries of Our Own Feelings

Discussion thus far has focused on how the other person may interpret our actions and choices of expression. But attentiveness to our own feelings is important as well. Sometimes an important reason for referral is our own attraction to someone who has come for help. When too powerful, such feelings can contaminate the ability to maintain appropriate distance and a calm presence. In fact, a pastor's poor handling of personal feelings may further complicate the struggle of a person already confused about who to trust.

One way to maintain a check on personal feelings is to examine regularly the areas already discussed in this section. It is time to look hard at ourselves if we: suggest, or are strongly inclined to suggest, meetings at a "cozy restaurant" for lunch instead of at the office; offer regularly to meet late in the afternoon after everyone else is gone; speak more frequently of our affection and regard for the person; consciously or inadvertently look for excuses to make physical contact. When we become aware of such feelings, it is important to start setting clear limits—on ourselves.

Summary

If you are wondering if the author is being a bit paranoid about all this, you are right! Anyone who believes in the doctrine of original sin has to be a bit paranoid—and rightly so. We human beings have all sorts of motives and desires. That is why you have been invited to look hard at these elements inside yourself. All of us are prone to confuse our roles and relationships. When that happens, the opportunity for genuine and helpful caring is severely compromised, and people are likely to be hurt. The bottom line here is this: beware of yourself and beware of others. Even when initiated without conscious intent of harm, caring relationships involve risk. That is normal, and if there were not some risk there would be less caring. Acknowledge the risk and watch for warning signs that things are getting out of hand. When you see them, heed them— for your well-being and for that of the person in your care.

Referral

The variety of sexual issues that come to a pastor's attention are complex and often call for specific knowledge with regard to treatment. It is also true that some problems respond positively to sensitive, well-managed pastoral support. In the chapters that follow, suggestions will be made to assist in sorting out the variables that apply in each case. However, it is important to emphasize that the process of referral itself can be an exceedingly significant event for the person.

Referral Reflects Our Own Willingness to Evaluate Ourselves

Contrary to the frequent fear that people will see a referral to someone else as an attempt to "get rid of" them, it is often the case that persons appreciate the willingness of a pastor to acknowledge what she or he can and cannot do. In fact, the very act of referral, if done well, can be a model for the process of self-evaluation. If we are willing to admit our limits (our finitude), then others are encouraged to admit their own.

Ability

Limits, of course, come in many varieties. The most obvious is that of training and ability. When we perceive that a person is struggling with something that is beyond our own understanding or training, then to refer is an act of being responsible. In an urban area in which there are many specialists, referral can be done with greater ease, of course. Rural areas may pose more problems in terms of professional availability and distance. Suggestions about appropriate specialists for referral will be made in the following chapters. However, the importance of referral is not diminished when such resources are relatively less available.

Several years ago the Menninger Clinic conducted a study of sources of stress, anxiety, and burnout among clergy (reported by Charles Rassieur in *Stress Management for Ministers*; Philadelphia: Westminster Press, 1982). One of the primary categories identified by the research team was named "imprecise competence"— their term for "flying by the seat of your pants." The investigators found that many ministers, because the community lacked other professionals or parishioners were unable to pay, attempted to work with problems for which they had little or no training. Their intentions, of course, were admirable. However, the result was ineffective at best and sometimes harmful.

In the absence of resources, in terms of either the minister's training or the parishioner's financial means, the most responsible thing for a minister to do is acknowledge, at the outset, his or her lack of special skills for dealing with the problem. This does not mean that listening and empathy, along with ongoing encouragement, cannot be offered, but no suggestion should be made that "treatment" is being rendered. To make such a promise, even indirectly, invites unrealistic hopes and may even discourage the person from seeking more specific help while receiving general pastoral support.

Time

There also are occasions in which a pastor may be confident in terms of ability but limited in terms of available time. Lack of time is just as important a reason as lack of ability to make a referral. This is true in general, but it is particularly true when dealing with sexual issues.

Persons struggling with sexual problems are acutely sensitive to rejection. Out of their own sensitivity, fear, or embarrassment, they are likely to interpret even slight indications of avoidance as negative judgments on them and their deeply embedded concerns. The opinions or responses of pastors or members of religious communities are likely to carry even more weight because

of the counselee's anxiety about theological disapproval or condemnation. In the midst of all those dynamics, promises of help
are taken very seriously.

Frequent changes of meeting times for otherwise perfectly
understandable reasons can be frustrating or even painful for the
parishioner who counts on pastoral time and presence. The time
between infrequently scheduled conversations can seem inter-
minable when emotional intensity is involved.

Therefore, if time is limited, a busy liturgical season is coming up, or a vacation or study leave is not far away, it is important
to refer rather than squeeze one more commitment into an already overloaded schedule. To refer under such circumstances is
vital for the pastor's own care of self and to avoid leading a person into thinking the pastor is more available than is realistic.
When a referral is made, however, it is still important to be available in a limited way for general pastoral support.

Referral Reflects the Importance
of Using the Larger Community

A discussion of ability and time necessarily focuses on the
pastor him- or herself. There is, however, another perspective to
be considered that has more general import. The pastor who seldom refers and attempts regularly to take on too much delivers
the subtle (and somewhat arrogant) message that the pastor is the
only credible resource. Put in therapeutic terms, such a style fosters overdependency. Put theologically, this style communicates a
lack of belief in the doctrine of the priesthood of all believers.

In fact, there are *many* people who can be of support to people struggling with painful issues, including sexual ones. A pastor
will contribute much by heightening a congregation's and individual parishioners' awareness of the many people in the community who are concerned and skilled. Some of those resource
people are professionals, but there are also trustworthy lay people
who have years of experience and sensitivity to offer through support groups and special friendships along the way.

An important pastoral responsibility is to know these people in the wider community and offer what Wayne Oates has called a "ministry of introduction." Such introductions are not only more realistic in terms of available time and ability, but they also provide assurance that the wider community is more gracious and caring than a suffering person might have believed. To become aware of wider resources and places to experience a community's concern is itself a part of the healing process. To contribute to a belief that only the pastor can be trusted fosters greater insecurity and thus impedes the healing process.

The Process of Referral

Referral is itself a teaching process. As noted above, the pastor's willingness to refer models the importance of acknowledging personal limits—an important lesson for persons wrestling with sexual expectations and disappointments. The identification of other resources within the community is also instructive; it widens awareness of the array of helpful sources for caring and healing that are all around us.

Explanation

Never make a referral without offering a clear explanation for doing so. If the reason is limited time, say so. If you feel unsure of your ability to work effectively with the issues involved, say so. If you feel reasonably confident but you know of someone who is more effective in dealing with this particular issue, say so. The most important part of explanation is openness, which discourages suspicion or concern about rejection in the person being referred.

The explanation should include not only reasons for making the referral but also the pastor's perception of the issues and perspectives that need attention in the new caring relationship being recommended. Describe the strengths that you see in the person that he or she can use for coping with difficulties. Note the places of difficulty you hope will be faced openly and willingly. In other words, tell all you know about your reasons and your hopes for the person's growth. Openness is crucial for the maintenance of trust.

Introduction

There are two important ingredients in introducing the referral source. The first is providing a sketch of who the person is and why she or he is considered a good choice. Often it is helpful to suggest two or three possibilities, allowing a range of options. The verbal portrait of the person should include personal as well as professional characteristics. Describe him or her in terms of age, gender, years of experience, approach or style, any particular reasons for trusting him or her, and experiences that illustrate such trustworthiness.

The second part of the introduction is to tell the person what you intend to say when calling to make the referral. After all, you are passing on personal information, and, again, it is a sign of trust and candor; no secrets are being kept about what you will say. In fact, this should be fairly easy to do, because a great deal of detail is not necessary when making a referral.

A description might go something like this: "I will call Dr. Jones and see about the possibilities for working with you. My only description will be to say you have been married for twenty-five years, have raised three children, have been reasonably happy until the last year, when you began experiencing difficulties in your sexual relationship. Now, you want to work on it. Unless you want me to say more, I think it will be best for you to fill in the details when you call to make your first appointment or in the first session."

The crucial element, again, is openness about what will be said. Your candor encourages the candor and trust of the person you are referring when he or she goes to meet and work with the new person.

Summary

Referral is far more than "passing someone on" for help. It is a significant teaching event that contributes to or impedes the healing process. Through disclosure of your own limits, open sharing of your motives and hopes, and candor about all that goes on in making the referral, you instill trust and offer hope.

One other important part of the referral process is walking the thin line between not doing enough and doing too much. While you should offer the important information about referral resources and also offer to make contact with the referral source on the parishioner's behalf, it is very important that the person make the first appointment personally. If the pastor does too much, the parishioner has little or no emotional investment in the process. That difficult act of picking up the telephone to make the appointment is an important step along the pilgrimage of growth.

Last, but not least, it is important to be *less* available in some ways to people after they have been referred. This, too, can be tricky. Making and receiving phone calls to talk about "how things are going" is a good thing, but to begin talking too specifically about what is going on in treatment sets up a divided loyalty. In this situation people may use pastoral support to deflect tough issues that need to be confronted with the professional they are seeing. If asked what you think about what the therapist or doctor said, it is wise to gently skirt the issue by encouraging the person to discuss it in treatment. Though such a response may be resented at first, it will be appreciated in the long run. If you are genuinely concerned and think you should become involved, openness and candor remain important. Offer to meet with the person *and* the therapist. Do not become a conduit through which therapist and client pass messages back and forth to each other. To do so may be to help the parishioner avoid direct communication.

Moving On

We have explored issues of self-awareness, sources of gender identity and their impact on sense of self, and important issues for the maintenance of a good pastoral relationship. The second part of this book will focus on particular sexual difficulties and ways in which we can respond with appropriate pastoral care.

For Further Reading

Two books published specifically on referral are William Oglesby's revised edition of *Referral in Pastoral Counseling* (Nashville: Abingdon Press, 1978), and the revised and enlarged edition of *Where to Go for Help*, by Wayne E. Oates and Kirk H. Neely (Philadelphia: Westminster Press, 1972). Although the resources they suggest are somewhat dated, both books are quite clear and helpful in the principles described.

The books suggested below are primarily general texts in pastoral care and counseling. In them you will find sections that deal with the concerns of this chapter: setting context and assuring a "safe place," pastoral conduct in the pastoral relationship, and referral.

Browning, Don S. *The Moral Context of Pastoral Care.* Philadelphia: Westminster Press, 1976.

———. *Religious Ethics and Pastoral Care.* Philadelphia: Fortress Press, 1983.

Childs, Brian. *Short-Term Pastoral Counseling: A Guide.* Nashville: Abingdon Press, 1990.

Clinebell, Howard. *Basic Types of Pastoral Care and Counseling: Resources for the Ministry of Healing and Growth.* Revised and enlarged. Nashville: Abingdon Press, 1984.

Cobb, John. *Theology and Pastoral Care.* Philadelpia: Fortress Press, 1977.

Friedman, Edwin H. *Generation to Generation: Family Process in Church and Synagogue.* New York: Guilford Press, 1985.

Hunter, Rodney J., ed. *Dictionary of Pastoral Care and Counseling.* Nashville: Abingdon Press, 1990.

Miller, William R., and Kathleen A. Jackson. *Practical Psychology for Pastors.* Englewood Cliffs, N.J.: Prentice-Hall, 1985.

Oates, Wayne E. *The Christian Pastor.* 3d ed. Philadelphia: Westminster Press, 1982.

———. *Pastoral Counseling.* Philadelphia: Westminster Press, 1974.

Rassieur, Charles L. *Stress Management for Ministers*. Philadelphia: Westminster Press, 1982.

The following list provides the names of several resources that deal specifically with pastoral care and the dangers of sexual impropriety.

Carlson, Robert J. "Battling Sexual Indiscretion." *Ministry*, January 1987, pp. 4–6.

Fortune, Marie. *Is Nothing Sacred: When Sex Invades the Pastoral Relationship*. San Francisco: Harper & Row, 1989.

Gabbard, Glen O., ed. *Sexual Exploitation in Professional Relationships*. Washington, D.C.: American Psychiatric Press, 1989.

Lebacqz, Karen, and Ronald G. Barton. *Sex in the Parish*. Louisville, Ky.: Westminster/John Knox Press, 1991.

Rediger, Lloyd G. *Ministry and Sexuality: Cases, Counseling, and Care*. Minneapolis: Fortress Press, 1990.

Rutter, Peter. *Sex in the Forbidden Zone*. Los Angeles: Jeremy P. Tarcher, 1986.

Persons interested in specific material on codes of conduct and proposed processes for dealing with inappropriate professional conduct may want to order a packet titled "Clergy Ethics: Sexual Abuse with the Pastoral Relationship." It is for sale through the Center for Prevention of Sexual and Domestic Violence, 1914 N. 34th St., Ste. 105, Seattle, WA 98103.

Professional codes of conduct may also be obtained from any number of professional groups, such as those for physicians or therapists. Most church denominations now have codes of conduct established or in process.

PART 2

SEXUAL ISSUES AND PASTORAL CARE

4

Sexual Dysfunction in Marriage

Rare is the pastor who does not have people coming in to talk about marital issues. Usually one partner comes alone. However, the odds for reconciliation are often better when the two come together. At least there seems to be mutual motivation to clarify the issues and communicate about them. It is relatively certain that if there are problems in the marriage, some of them are disturbing the sexual relationship of the couple.

However, many people will not want to talk about sex, perhaps because it seems *too* concrete and physical and, of course, because it has always been difficult to talk about sex in a "churchy" environment. They may also think, "After all, if we straighten out everything else, sex will just fall into place." At one level, the assumption that all else will fall into place is true. If communication is going well, then sexual conflicts can be dealt with straightforwardly along with everything else. The problem is that resentments, fears, and expectations characterize the sexual relationship of any struggling couple. Their very resistance to discussing sex is both reflective of the poor job the church has done in dealing with sex in the past and symbolic of the difficulty the couple have discussing anything intimate with each other.

Furthermore, reluctance to talk about sexual matters is often an indication of relative ignorance about the theological, psychological, and physiological ways in which sexuality functions in a marriage. Uncomfortable though it may make the pastor, offering an invitation to make sex "speakable" is often helpful, if not essential. The intent, of course, is not to be voyeuristic about what a couple does. Rather, the aim is to affirm sexuality as one of a number of arenas that offer an opportunity for couples to learn to communicate and care for each other more openly and sensitively.

In this and the following chapters, we will explore the difficulties and possibilities for dealing with the particular issue in terms of several frames of reference. We will view sexual dysfunction in marriage from theological, psychological, and physiological perspectives. In these discussions communication will be examined as a major shaping influence in the movement toward either enriched intimacy or more painful dysfunction.

The Theological

In pastoral care, every minister faces the task of providing a theological perspective on the life issues with which people struggle. This does not necessarily mean getting into "God talk," although frequently that is just what is needed. Most important is that the clergyperson have a clear frame of reference to help guide the conversation. Guiding, of course, is not the same thing as controlling. In fact, a healthy theological frame of reference often helps the pastor maintain a listening stance instead of jumping in prematurely with unhelpful words of advice.

Sadly, many persons think that some subjects are not appropriate for a pastoral conversation. Sex is often one of those subjects. If the pastor has not thought about sexuality within his or her theological understanding of human nature, then there will be awkwardness and hesitation about dealing with it. When both pastor *and* parishioners are uneasy, you can be sure that it will not be discussed!

One of the first things to bear in mind is that many people in the church today are victims of what has been called the "mind-body dualism," a radical (and artificial) separation of physical, or "earthly," matters from the "more important," or spiritual, issues. Such a view is expressed through what some writers have described as the spiritualizing of the church. This distorted perspective narrowly defines the spiritual dimensions of life with which pastors and church members should be concerned. More concrete and earthly matters are treated as out of bounds, even viewed as not important. The results of such thinking are unfortunate from several points of view.

One negative result is that people are often ashamed and embarrassed to admit that sexual issues "interfere" with their feelings for each other and with the sense of satisfaction they would like to have in their work, their daily activities, and even their participation in the life of the church. This sense of shame manifests itself in reluctance and discomfort when talking about intimacy of any kind.

The mind-body split generates internal messages that compound the problem. The inner voice says, "Don't bother the minister with that." "If you'll just get a grip on yourself, then things will work out." "Sex isn't something you talk about; you just *do it!*"

An important biblical and theological message is ignored, or at least minimized, in such thinking. When God created the world, *everything* in it was pronounced good. Creation theology, often neglected in our day because of the very dualism discussed above, reminds us that the *earth* and all that is in it are the Lord's. Therefore, earthly things and the activities of our daily life are intended to be pleasing and fulfilling to both God and humankind. For creation to function at its best, and for human beings to experience the richness that God intended, the spirit and the flesh cannot be artificially separated. Such a separation inevitably results in the labeling of one side of the division as good and the other side as bad, even evil.

Some of the most rigid puritanical thinking comes out of the division between things of the spirit and "things of the world." The obvious intent is to guard against irresponsible behavior, sexual and otherwise. However, just the reverse is often accomplished. In fact, "the flesh" is most likely to get into trouble and cause the greatest pain when it is artificially separated from the spirit that shapes and gives expression to beauty through our incarnation. Without the vital union between the various dimensions of the self, alienation and human suffering become more likely. When the union of mind, body, and spirit is acknowledged and preserved, it is far more likely that responsible, committed, and enriching sexual behavior will result.

When two people are committed to an intimate relationship in marriage but have difficulty talking to each other about the basic elements of their existence together, then a damaging separation between the spirit and the flesh has taken place. Interestingly, the result is that they have trouble talking about deeper spiritual issues as well as sexual behavior. On the other hand, do not assume that only sex is hard to talk about. It will also be difficult to differ in a way that is sensitive and understanding over who pays the bills or who sees to the maintenance of the car.

To move people into talking about sexual issues may evoke greater seriousness and focus than rehashing the problems with the checking account. This happens because issues of sexuality lie near the heart of what it means to love and be loved *fully*—heart and soul, body and mind.

Reinhold Niebuhr helped us to see this vital connection in his discussions of human nature (see *The Nature and Destiny of Man*, vol. 1). One helpful description drawn from Niebuhr's discussion is to say that we are a blending of body and mind, animated by spirit. As have so many other theologians, he was seeking to describe the integrated nature of human be-ing. Body, mind, and spirit are inseparably linked by God's creative work. However, we human beings have a hard time living with the creative tension that results from the unification of these expressions of who we are.

Human beings are complex, and anxiety grows out of our awareness of what complicated creatures we are. The mind can imagine and desire things far beyond the ability of the body. The body is subject to all sorts of inexplicable urges and sensations. The spirit guides the body and the mind in finding workable, cooperative, and sometimes surprising ways of living with this integral connectedness of the various dimensions of our selves, but often it is difficult to distinguish the promptings of the spirit from other urges and desires. Being human is difficult and anxiety-laden.

Anxiety, said Niebuhr, is also the breeding ground for sin. Thus, we might extrapolate that in our discomfort with anxiety, with not fully understanding ourselves, with not being able to be completely in control of our lives, we seek a simplified order by ignoring or even demeaning parts of ourselves or others. Rather than acknowledging fantasies and expectations with regard to sex, for example, one may act as if sex does not matter. Rather than admitting ignorance about how best to excite and delight a partner, a spouse may pretend to know and then become angry if the partner does not enjoy it. Rather than seek to find the ways to give and take, love and be loved through communication, one may avoid talking about what matters most.

When two people have not talked about sex, or have become inordinately angry with each other for not satisfying sexual needs, they have fallen into one expression of what Niebuhr would probably describe as sin. By not talking with each other, they are refusing to acknowledge their human need for each other. Their failure to understand this is in part a consequence of poor education about who they are as children of God.

In light of the racy stories that circulate about sexual expression in our day, the following case may seem dull and out of date. But it is not. In our fascination with the dramatic, we often overlook far more common situations like this one.

George and Nancy came to talk to their minister about the ongoing unhappiness in their thirty-year marriage. He was sixty, she fifty-eight. Nancy did most of the talking. She described her increasing frustration with George when he came home in the evenings. Routinely she prepared a warm meal, took a shower just before he arrived home, and mentally coached herself to ask about his day before telling him about hers. In many ways, she still sought to be the "good wife." And George was a good provider, but was always tired when he got home. He would ignore Nancy's attempted kiss as he came through the door, heading immediately to the den to watch television until she called him to the dinner table. Even then, he often picked up his plate from the already set table and carried it back to the den, where he would eat by himself while Nancy cried or banged dishes in the kitchen.

George did not disagree with anything Nancy did or said. He insisted that he *really was* tired when he came home. Why couldn't she understand that? He provided a good living for her. She was free to pursue her interests during the day. He had never been unfaithful. Weren't these things proof enough of his love? What more could she want?

Stereotypical as this may sound, the dynamics are real for many marriages. Hopes and dreams are seldom discussed. Unspoken assumptions are made about what the other person wants or deserves. In this case, the pastor made numerous attempts to help their communication, inviting Nancy to tell George more of what she wanted from the marriage. In the first session it was clear that George knew of all the preparations Nancy made each day for his returning home. He was consciously ignoring them! To the pastor, this seemed an opportunity for encouraging them to tell each other more about their hopes and dreams for a shared life—talking more, doing more things together, finding a rhythm for respecting each other's need for privacy and rest, and more. However, even though both faithfully came to the several sessions with their pastor, no observable improvement was noted in their relationship.

In what was more an attempt born of desperation than a skilled and calculated move, the pastor finally inquired about their sexual relationship. Her question was one of several attempting to identify positive dimensions of their life together. At first there was silence, then Nancy began to speak, haltingly and with embarrassment. She said she missed sex and described her sadness that George obviously didn't find her attractive. She was feeling terribly rejected by George and wondered what was "wrong" with her that "turned him off."

George looked at her with surprise and began to speak haltingly of his sense of shame and embarrassment that he couldn't count on getting an erection. In addition, he was feeling sensitive about his baldness and his expanding waistline. He had become convinced that he was no longer sexually attractive to *her*. So, he found regular excuses (like being tired) to avoid the anticipated embarrassment or rejection.

Had they ever talked about this before? No. When they had gone to a pastor for premarital education, they had been asked about their hopes for the sexual dimension of their marriage. They had avoided talking about it then, and the minister had seemed relieved. After all, they weren't married yet, and they felt guilty at the thought of telling the pastor they had been having intercourse throughout their dating relationship, even though they were fairly sure that the minister knew.

George and Nancy's pattern of not talking about uncomfortable matters had become a habit. As a matter of fact, they did not think their parents had really talked to each other about troublesome issues. Furthermore, they both were operating on the assumption that the sexual relationship was something that should not be talked about. It was something that people should just know how to handle, an activity to be hidden first from a pastor and now from each other. A distorted understanding of Christian faith was partially informing their sense that sexual issues should not be that important (except negatively!) and should not receive undue attention. At the same time, they both had deep concerns about their relationship because of disappointments growing out of their unshared fears and wishes. They were rapidly moving toward what amounted to no more than a sense of obligation to remain with each other. The commitment seemed increasingly a matter of the will and not also of the heart.

A dualistic theology, though unrecognized by them, had contributed significantly to their present problems. Nancy had learned that sex was a duty. You just "do it" without discussing it. George had learned that sex was only a matter of physical attraction, thus separate from other thoughts and feelings. They had been careful to avoid speaking of their fears about their sexual relationship with each other and thus had unwittingly missed the growth, exploration, and joy that could come from seeing *all* things as part of God's good creation. Cultivating the ability to talk about intimacy would have contributed to their effectiveness in working through their problems, to discovering relatively simple physiological and emotional facts that could help them.

A mind-body dualism had cut them off from seeing the importance of talking about these very basic issues in their life together. The absence of those conversations thus deprived them of deeper forms of sharing.

Now, after all these years, as they sat with a minister in a religious setting again, the sexual relationship became the context within which they could begin to talk about their fears and their hopes for the first time. The very intensity of the subject, and the discomfort they felt, got their attention more effectively than simply reviewing the things they had already talked about over and over again. They now had a pastor who carefully and sensitively began to talk with them about the care and joy, rather than fear and duty, with which they were called to love each other.

Hard as it may be to believe, Nancy and George were separated from each other because of an unarticulated and artificial theological "message" that subtly dominated their thinking and thus their behavior. One manifestation of that dualism was their lack of awareness of the importance and need even to talk about matters of intimacy, followed by their discomfort with doing so once the need was seen. Any pastor would do well to be aware of this theological contribution to problems in intimacy.

The Psychological

We have considered some origins of discomfort for marital partners in developing sexual intimacy from a theological perspective. Now, we will turn our attention to some of the psychological dimensions involved in sexual dysfunction.

Let's look at another example. Martha and Christopher illustrate some basic communication issues that get in the way of people enjoying their sexual relationship. When difficulties first became apparent, Martha stated her desire to learn more about what Christopher wanted her to do when they engaged in love-making and intercourse. In like manner, she wanted to tell him of her needs and desires. Christopher, on the other hand, said he resented her "trying to tell me what to do." Despite her protests that it was not her intent to give him "directions," Christopher could not hear it any other way.

What is going on between them? Of many psychological issues that could be discussed, we will focus on ongoing studies about gender differences.

Because no one person fits all these characteristics, we must be careful about making premature assumptions about a particular man or woman. However, there is a great deal of recent research, referred to briefly in chapter 2, that does alert us to watch for certain communication patterns related to gender.

For example, the bulk of the literature on gender characteristics notes that females are generally more inclined toward behavior that promotes equality, harmony, and understanding. In pursuit of these purposes (which many neurobiologists would say conform to their brain structure), women will be alert to a variety of signals, options, and possibilities for bringing about these goals. They will also be prone to assume that their intention is shared by all concerned. If married, that assumption is especially true with regard to a husband.

Martha reflects that general profile in her desire to share information with Christopher. Her goal is to promote greater mutual enjoyment of their lovemaking. In carrying out that task, which she was sure that Christopher would appreciate, she gave him knowledge about herself and her desires—what "turned her on." Telling him those things about herself was largely, for her, an act of intimacy and vulnerability. For Christopher to respond with hostility was confusing to her, and hurtful. The only obvious conclusion that she could draw was that he did not want to be intimate, to be responsive to her, or even to accept her initiatives toward him. From the point of view of one who seeks harmony, her conclusion was perfectly understandable. The same dynamic is manifested in our earlier case. Nancy's preparations before

71

George came home were also oriented toward mutuality, intimacy, and sharing.

Let us quickly say that these examples are not intended to promote the idea that females are naturally oriented toward becoming the stereotypical "total woman." The point is that there seems to be an orientation on the part of the "average" female toward intimacy, connection, symmetry, and community. Certainly there are females who are exceptions to this, and they are no less human and certainly no less female. They simply do not represent as fully the findings on typical "femaleness" that are reflected in current studies.

It is also important to say here that the outcome of gender research is not intended to generate prescriptive definitions of masculinity and femininity. Normative statements, as presented here, are not value judgments that demand conformity. Rather, these findings contribute to the search for general patterns that may contribute to the misunderstanding that appears in so many male-female relationships. With those caveats, we will return to the case of Martha and Christopher.

Christopher reflects the normative male who appears in recent gender studies. In the face of Martha's suggestions for a way of enriching their love life, he perceives that she is attempting to control the relationship. That perception is more likely a reflection of what is going on within himself than what is going on within her. Inclined to think more hierarchically, a male often hears a suggestion or unsolicited information as an attempt by the other person to be "one-up," as a competitive suggestion that there is something he does not know. The typical male response to such perceived competition is to demonstrate that he already knows it or that the information is not important anyway. If successful in this self-generated contest, the male retains what seems more important to him—independence and the avoidance of perceived failure or ignorance.

Now, it is indeed and in fact true that Martha knows something that Christopher does not—how *she* feels and what *she* prefers in lovemaking. The problem occurs at the point of how he will feel and react in the face of not knowing what she knows. Martha, as a normative female, is willing to acknowledge what she does not know and to learn about Christopher for the sake of the relationship. Christopher does not want Martha to know what he does not know—in order to preserve his own sense of competence—for the sake of the relationship. Unlike the female, key orientations for the normative male include independence, status, asymmetry, and contest.

With Martha and Christopher, as well as with George and Nancy, some key pastoral work can take place around helping them to understand these differences. Not only is it important to clarify the dissimilarities, but it is equally important to assure each that the characteristics are not personally directed against the other. In fact, each has admirable motivation that, if understood, can enrich the relationship. Furthermore, the disparity is characteristic of the genders, not of just these two persons. Once these variations are understood and accepted as givens, there should be less tendency for each to "take it personally."

Psychotherapists have a vocabulary that helps to describe this promotion of understanding. One term is to "reframe" the differences—to help them to be seen differently, in a more positive framework. They can be seen as strengths rather than problems—as evidence of "normality," rather than huge, exaggerated, unique faults that render people somehow "defective" as individuals or as a couple. Other terms used to describe the process of reassurance are "normalize" and "universalize," again helping the couple to see that their differences are a part of normal human life, typically shared by men and women across the board. With that knowledge, a couple can devote their time and energy to acceptance and understanding of these differences and finding ways either to sidestep them or find opportunities for growth in them.

The Physiological

Along with the theological and psychological issues discussed thus far, a pastor needs to be reminded that there are also very real physiological factors that play a role in sexual dysfunction. The work in recent decades of people like Masters and Johnson, Zilbergeld, Lonnie Barbach, and Helen Singer Kaplan have shown us just how much we do not know about our bodies. This is particularly true of the ways in which we function sexually.

For example, George, whom we met earlier in this chapter, can now accept and understand the negative effect of theological dualism on his sexual relationship with Nancy. Further, he can learn to communicate more openly about his fears and his preferences. However, he still may find that he has difficulty in getting and maintaining an erection—even when he is attracted to Nancy and wants to make love. It can be a matter of genuine relief for him to know that it is typical for males during and after midlife to need more manual stimulation to get and maintain an erection. That does not have to be bad news. It can even make for enjoyable and prolonged lovemaking.

In like manner, a woman needs to know that pain or discomfort during sexual intercourse may be due to vaginal dryness. The dryness is a physiological fact that increases with age and may have little to do with whether she is attracted to the man. There are a variety of vaginal creams and lubricants that are easy to use and can provide pleasure for both her and her partner.

Similar bits of information about both male and female physiology and sexual functioning can be enlightening and liberating to women and men alike. In fact, a shared process of learning more about their respective physiologies can be a major contributor to care of self, care of the partner, and care of the relationship and their enjoyment of it.

Men and women often find themselves avoiding lovemaking because reality does not meet the fantasies they have held about themselves and/or for their partner. Our culture has laid many exaggerated expectations on us in this so-called liberated era. In many ways, the liberation has made people slaves to commercialized standards for "success" that are physiologically unwise and often damaging.

Our bodies reflect much of what we have discussed theologically and psychologically. Genuinely intimate relationships are built. They do not just happen. There are phases in the cycle of sexual response with which, instead of trying to avoid or alter, we should cooperate: a period of excitement, followed by a plateau, followed by a rush of "orgasmic inevitability" culminating in orgasm, followed by a period of resolution. Much detail is now available about the characteristics of these stages, how to cooperate with them, and how to find rich enjoyment in each of them. Pastors should have at least a general knowledge about this information, but they should not expect themselves to become sex therapists.

A Word of Caution

A word needs to be said here about sex therapy, much of which is oriented toward teaching about these physiological characteristics of the sexual response cycle. A number of techniques are now available that have very impressive rates of success. Many of them are variations and refinements of the work published by Masters and Johnson, who first received major public attention for sex therapy. The techniques involve a set of progressive exercises that involve getting to know one's own and one's partner's body. The steps in the process must be taken deliberately and without hurry. Many of the failures in sex therapy are a result of inappropriately pressuring a couple to move prematurely beyond their developing levels of comfort and acceptance of what is being learned.

While these exercises are simple, my recommendation to any pastor is: *Do not attempt to use these approaches unless you have been specifically trained or unless you are under skilled supervision!* If an approach is used awkwardly or insensitively, it will be more difficult for a skilled therapist to effectively use the process later, because it will have been contaminated in its earlier introduction.

Pastoral Practice

The task of the pastor in general is to use the principles outlined in chapter 3. Specific suggestions are offered here for the pastor working with couples who are troubled and uncertain about their sexual relationship.

First, after hearing the anguish of these people, *encourage* them by offering a theological perspective that accepts these problems as normal for the human condition. Part of our finitude (not sin!) as human beings is that we are sensitive and fearful when we face the possibility of genuine intimacy with each other. Our finitude often is reflected in our ignorance and our fear of admitting it. Just as we are invited into a process of coming to know God, even when it is anxiety-producing, we are invited into such a process with each other. To deal with our sexual relationship is to be faithful to God's intentions for humankind. God takes our down-to-earth passions and desires just as seriously as our spiritual journeys. In discussing these matters, judicious use of vocabulary is important, of course; take into account where these people are in their spiritual understanding and comfort.

Second, offer a psychological perspective on what is happening. Inform partners that they may be struggling with some of the differences between men and women. Teach them ways in which they can learn from each other and develop communication habits that will strengthen them as individuals and as a couple.

Third, *talk about sex without apology*. Let them know that their bodies are important to God. After all, we are told even in the New Testament that our bodies are temples for the Holy Spirit (see 1 Cor. 6:19–20). Marital partners have the enjoyable responsibility of learning about their bodies for the glorification of God through their faithfulness to each other and through the ecstasy and abandon that can come from discovering more about how we are created and how we can love each other.

Fourth, if it seems wise based on our discussion in chapter 3, *make a good referral* to a certified sex therapist to help partners work through particularly difficult and prolonged problems. More and more psychiatrists, psychologists, clinical social workers, and pastoral counselors are trained in these techniques. Remember to ask specifically about a professional person's training before making referrals to him or her. If you are near a university medical school, call and ask for the names of people regarded as adequately trained. Try to get to know a trained sex therapist so that you can refer to him or her with confidence.

The richness these couples gain in their sexual relationships will energize them for fuller service to God and the wider world in which they live.

For Further Reading

To explore some of the theological frames of reference further, I recommend a reading of Reinhold Niebuhr's *The Nature and Destiny of Man*, volume I in particular (New York: Charles Scribner's Sons, 1941; reprinted 1964). A rereading of your own favorite theologian's doctrine of human nature will be helpful when done with sexuality as the chief concern. However, neither Niebuhr nor many of the classical systematic theologians deal at length with sexual issues, so further attention could well be given to some writers who have specialized in this subject. One of the most helpful is James B. Nelson in *Embodiment: An Approach to Sexuality and Christian Theology* (Minneapolis: Augsburg Publishing House, 1978) and his more recent *Body Theology* (Louisville, Ky.: Westminster/John Knox Press, 1992). See the bibliographical suggestions at the end of chapter 2 for other resources of this sort.

For readings on some of the psychological and neurological differences between women and men, I recommend again the works of Moir and Tannen, noted at the end of chapter 2.

A number of helpful works give particular attention to the matter of sexual dysfunction. Perhaps the most comprehensive are those written by Masters and Johnson and Helen Singer Kaplan. The reader willing to devote the time needed for a thorough reading will learn a great deal about the human body and its sexual functioning from *Human Sexual Response*, by William H. Masters and Virginia E. Johnson (Boston: Little, Brown & Co., 1966). Masters and Johnson deal specifically with sexual dysfunction and its treatment in their later work, *Human Sexual Inadequacy* (Boston: Little, Brown & Co., 1970). Helen Singer

Kaplan consistently provides information both about the body and its sexual functioning and the treatment of various dysfunctions in *Disorders of Sexual Desire and Other New Concepts and Techniques in Sex Therapy* (New York: Simon & Schuster, 1979) and *The New Sex Therapy: Active Treatment of Sexual Dysfunctions* (New York: Brunner/Mazel, 1981). Another comprehensive work is *Treatment of Sexual Dysfunction: A Bio-Psycho-Social Approach* by William E. Hartman and Marilyn A. Fithian (Arcadia, N.Y.: Aronson, 1974).

Many less technical books are available and useful to pastors and parishioners in their quest to learn more about sexual functioning and ways to enhance enjoyment including prescribed steps for working on problems of dysfunction. Note that there are books devoted to female, male, and couple issues.

Barbach, Lonnie. *For Each Other: Sharing Sexual Intimacy*. New York: Doubleday, Anchor Books, 1982.
———. *For Yourself: The Fulfillment of Female Sexuality*. New York: Doubleday, Anchor Books, 1975.
Knopf, Jennifer, and Michael Seiler. *ISD: Inhibited Sexual Desire*. New York: William Morrow & Co., 1990.
Zilbergeld, Bernie. *Male Sexuality*. New York: Bantam Books, 1978.

Several books are suggested for the pastor's own reflection about approaches to working with couples. *Reframing*, by Donald Capps (Philadelphia: Fortress Press, 1990), is not tied specifically to sexual issues but introduces further the concept of "reframing," mentioned in this chapter.

Several works also useful for pastoral care and counseling on sexual issues as such follow.

Kennedy, Eugene. *Sexual Counseling*. San Francisco: Seabury Press, 1977.
Mace, David R. *Sexual Difficulties in Marriage*. Philadelphia: Fortress Press, 1972.

Rice, Philip. *Sexual Problems in Marriage: Help from a Christian Counselor*. Philadelphia: Westminster Press, 1978.

A more comprehensive book that pulls together perspectives from several disciplines is *Integrating Sex and Marital Therapy*, edited by Gerald R. Weeks and Larry Hof (New York: Brunner/Mazel, 1987). Hof is himself theologically trained.

Finally, it is helpful for a pastor to have several technical and pictorial manuals to lend to persons dealing with sexual dysfunction. I recommend *The Joy of Sex*, edited by Alex Comfort (New York: Simon & Schuster, 1972). Although the book was considered "shocking" when it first appeared, it also is open in its willingness to encourage experimenting with various techniques in lovemaking. For some marital partners, it becomes a device for getting permission to explore new opportunities for romance. If that book is too discomforting for some people, a more clinical but equally specific manual is *The Illustrated Manual of Sex Therapy* by Helen Singer Kaplan (New York: Quadrangle/The New York Times Book Company, 1972). This manual is tied to her book *The New Sex Therapy*, mentioned above.

It is very important that a pastor *not* suggest any of these books without having read them first. Remember that recommendation is interpreted by most to imply agreement with what is said in it and willingness to discuss any of its content. Again, your level of self-awareness and comfort should dictate what you recommend. To suggest the book and later be unwilling to discuss the reading or shocked at conversations prompted by it reinforces the sexual dualism that needs rather to be undermined.

5
Extramarital Affairs

In modern-day life, as in the Bible, extramarital affairs are mentioned frequently. Both popular magazines and careful research report troubling statistics on marital infidelity. Serious problems are evident. But what exactly *are* the problems? Where should pastoral energy be focused in the face of confessions, accusations, and rumors in congregations and the wider community? How does one respond to situations such as the following?

Jane, married to Herbert for thirty years, weeps softly in her pastor's study. As the result of a stroke, Herbert has been bedridden and in a nursing home for the last nine years. Jane has been seeing Bob for a year now and is finding the deep companionship that she desperately wants. "I can't divorce Herbert," she says. "If I did that when he is so helpless, the guilt would kill me. It's unusual, I know, but what's really wrong with my just having a long-term affair with Bob? He understands and is willing. In fact, the relationship with Bob would probably help me care for Herbert with less resentment."

"She just got more and more boring," says Walter of Marion, his wife of twenty-five years. "She invested her whole life in the children, and I became no more than the moneymaker she needed to care for them. So I found someone who loved *me*. If Marion doesn't like it, tough. It's her own fault."

Jim shifts uncomfortably in his chair, takes a deep breath, and says, "Thanks for telling me that the nominating committee would like me to serve as a deacon. I'm honored. But, I can't do it. As you know, this is my second marriage. What you may not know is that my present wife and I had an affair and finally ended both of our first marriages in order to be together. That was a long time ago—ten years, as a matter of fact. But you wouldn't want to let someone like me be a church officer, would you?"

"Pastor, I think my son is having an affair with his old college sweetheart. How do I know? Well, every time I visit him and his wife, she looks teary and worn out. He isn't around home with her very much. And my friends have told me they see him at lunch with his old flame on a regular basis. Every once in a while he mutters something about having married too young. Would you talk to him?"

"Pastor, I'm convinced she's having an affair. She meets with him every day after work. They talk on the phone every weekend, whether we are in town or away. But she says they are just very close—not having sex—just very close. But it sure feels like an affair to me."

What is going on in each of these situations? While the problem of affairs is common to each, the circumstances, motivations, and needs are not the same. The feelings that draw people together and drive them apart are complicated. Even defining an affair is complex. Take the last example, for instance. If the man's wife and her "friend" are not having sexual intercourse, can they be accused of having an affair? We will look at some of the dynamics of extramarital affairs from several perspectives.

The Theological

Even a cursory reading of the Bible, particularly the Old Testament, yields multiple examples of what we in our own day would describe as marital sexual infidelity. Yet the attitude and involvement of God varies significantly from case to case.

Careful analysis is needed to identify and evaluate the factors that come into play. For example, in Genesis 16 we are told that Abram is asked by his wife, Sarai, to "go in to" Hagar. Sarai is barren, and she wants their marriage to have a child—a very important issue in the Old Testament. Extramarital sex certainly takes place in this story, but it is at the request of the wife to serve the particular function of having a child. The controlling value here is not adultery but the priority of having children. Other values, even sexual involvement with another person, are secondary here. Abram's sexual activity with Hagar was done "for the sake of" his marriage with Sarai.

There may even be some parallels here to situations in our own time, such as using sperm donors or surrogate mothers (personally or through a laboratory) to bring children to a barren marriage. For that matter, it is not uncommon for a single man or woman to wish for a child but not a marriage. Hence, they solicit a partner to serve the function of fathering or mothering in order to bring about conception. On occasion that chosen "partner" is married to someone else. Litigation and legislation show that some of these modern-day situations later experience the same dynamic as did Sarai and Abram: Hagar looks "with contempt" at Sarai after Hagar gives birth, Sarai orders her away, and Abram secretly arranges for Hagar's well-being. The point here is that extramarital sexual activity may take place to serve a function other than lust or infidelity. It must also be said that the Bible clearly shows the complications and injury that can take place within such an intimate realm.

In another illustration, the eleventh chapter of 2 Samuel records the story of David and Bathsheba. David, captivated by Bathsheba, has her brought to him so that he can "lie with her," even though he knows that she is married to Uriah. Later, upon receiving word from her that she is pregnant, he sets forces into motion that lead to Uriah's death, and to his marriage to Bathsheba and the birth of their child. This was extramarital infidelity based on personal desire, and God punished David for it. The controlling value was lust rather than a desire for the well-being of marriage or parenthood, as in the case of Sarai and Abram.

The book of Hosea records God's directive to Hosea to marry a whore! Again, a function or value is being served. We just have to figure out what it is and how God seems to view it. Through Hosea's marriage to Gomer, the impact of Israel's infidelity to God is personified and made concrete. And, of equal importance, the availability of forgiveness is affirmed. The controlling value here seems to be the importance of responding to a direct call from God, no matter how radical. The use of a sexual context makes the message that much more graphic.

Many more examples of the joys and woes of family life are recorded in the Hebrew scriptures—many of them complicated by various forms of infidelity. By the time of the New Testament an evolution toward monogamy as a primary value in and of itself has taken place, reflecting both the decreasing need for progeny and a growing awareness of human nature and the complications of multiple intimate relationships. Paul's first letter to the Corinthians states quite clearly that "each man should have his own wife [singular] and each woman her own husband" (7:2). This exhortation reflects the admonition of the Old Testament commandment not to covet another person's spouse.

In our day, relatively little ire is raised about sperm solicitation or surrogate mothers. But the sexual revolution notwithstanding, jealousy, rage, and hurt are regular responses to an extramarital affair. Our biblical and theological roots, discussed earlier, give us some clues to the reasons.

As monogamy increasingly becomes the norm for marriage in scripture, it reflects the evolving human understanding of the importance of and reasons for monotheism. God is declared time and again to be *the* one God, not simply a god among gods. Neither religious devotion nor the marital covenant are feasible with multiple commitments. Commitment to another god is idolatry. Intimate commitment to a person other than one's marital partner is adultery.

Commitment to marital partners and to God are characterized by *jealous* devotion. Interestingly, powerful self-references are made by God to being jealous. Exodus 34:14 states that ". . . you shall worship no other god, because the LORD, *whose name is Jealous*, is a jealous God" (emphasis added). Jealousy here is not viewed as a negative or immature concept. Rather, in this context it is a declaration of absolute devotion. As deeper understanding of the nature of the marital relationship develops, marriage becomes a human expression for the absolute, jealous devotion expected by God. Two people are pledged to be intimate *only* with each other, just as human beings are called to be intimate and worshipful of *only* one God. Another way of describing such a relationship is to say that it demonstrates fidelity.

By our standards, women were treated poorly in the Old Testament world. Yet, in spite of women's relatively low status, it is interesting to note the high regard in which marriage was held. Marriage symbolized the covenant of devotion and fidelity that God extends to humanity. The levirate marriage (Deut. 25:5–10) was an illustration of the depth of ties formed by marriage between families. Monogamy, though not universal, was clearly the norm, as evidenced by the tenth commandment and other supporting texts in Leviticus (18:20) and Numbers (5:12–31). Even though in one sense women were not honored, marriage was.

Consider one further observation from scripture. In Luke 20:34–35, Jesus speaks of marriage as a structure of that particular age, perhaps implying that it is a necessary way to express and receive fidelity at a human level. It would be better, he goes on to say, if people did not marry so that they could have their fidelity and devotion more exclusively directed toward God. Is this another reflection of God's jealousy for our undiverted attention? It is at least an indication of the relative importance placed on the devotion of human beings to each other as compared to the devotion expected from them for God.

Scripture and the history of theology seldom have strayed from a strong affirmation of the importance of a marital relationship being undisturbed by infidelity. Fidelity is important for the well-being of children raised within its walls, for the avoidance of unnecessary conflict in the midst of our already stressful human existence, and as a testimony to the importance of our being similarly unwavering in our devotion to God. It is therefore no surprise that extramarital affairs are viewed with serious concern and even stern judgment.

At the same time, scripture and most theological traditions acknowledge the complexity of human life and the reality of sin and finitude. When extramarital affairs occur in scripture, although they may not receive approval, there seems to be no surprise that they take place. Note again the frequency with which such experiences are acknowledged, particularly in the Old Testament. The absence of approval does not seem to imply that there are not understandable phenomena that explain the behavior—they do not excuse the involvement, but they do explain it. It is also important to remember that when finitude and sin are acknowledged, the most important responses are understanding, exploration of the possibilities for growth rather than further harm, and finding ways to offer and receive forgiveness.

The reality of finitude—of running up against one's limits—calls for understanding of the human frailty that we all share. There are some things that we just cannot control or manage. Sin implies error, distortion, missing the mark. When pain is reflected through an extramarital affair, some corrective action or understanding needs to take place. When harm is done because of finitude or sin, one form of correction is confession: admitting to the limit or the wrongdoing. Forgiveness is another, and it is difficult, because at the human level it requires that the offended party both have respect for the offender's confession and acknowledge oneself as human and equally capable of coming up short or missing the mark. Only in the context of all parties "owning" their finitude and sin is there a possibility for reconciliation—a "coming together" of some kind. Reconciliation does not automatically imply restoration of the former relationship. It may be that so much damage has occurred or the limits are so profound or the sin is so unbridled that reconciliation takes the form of an agreement that the former relationship is not restorable. In such a case, reconciliation may mean a joint agreement on the necessity for separateness rather than togetherness.

The more we plumb these various possibilities, the more we recognize that scripture and theology can be amplified and clarified by turning to some of the human sciences. The clinical disciplines are articulate in sorting through events and naming some of the "beasts" in our human nature. So we will move now to a psychological perspective.

The Psychological

Psychological awareness can both assist in understanding and confront us with the complexity of such a sensitive and conflictual issue as extramarital affairs. This section will explore several frames of reference that can help us to understand some of what is going on. These viewpoints do not neatly exclude each other, of course. Rather, they help us look from several vantage points

One clarifying note should be made here. When extramarital affairs are discussed in the literature, the major focus is not so much on whether sexual contact of some kind has taken place as on the *emotional attachment* that has formed. Of course, sexual contact certainly intensifies emotional bonding, but strong attachments that result in "infidelity" to other relationships can exist without the additional element of physical involvement.

Family-of-Origin Issues

Interestingly enough, the oft-quoted verse Deuteronomy 5:9 expresses something of the psychology involved in family-of-origin theory. It refers to God's punishment of children to the third and fourth generations for their parents' iniquities. Children do pay a price for the modeling passed on intentionally and unintentionally by parents and other significant family figures. One of the common patterns "transmitted" is that of extramarital affairs. The family histories of persons involved in affairs often reveal patterns of infidelity in the previous generations. Family-of-origin research reveals that an affair can be a learned response to anxiety or conflict. When conflict is going on within a marriage, the most primitive responses of the psyche are to flee or fight. Of course, there are a variety of ways to run or attack. Literal, physical escapes or assaults are two options. An affair is another. In fact, an affair is a way of escaping and attacking at the same time.

It is literally "running away" to another person for understanding, excitement, diversion, or a "quick fix." At the same time, because of the psychological pain it inflicts, it is an attack on the marital partner. Interestingly enough, it may be the *only* response the person has "learned" from his or her family of origin: When a relationship is a source of pain and confusion, flee into the arms of another.

Before such an interpretation is dismissed as rationalization and excuse-making, bear in mind that many people have genuine deficits in learning when it comes to dealing with emotional situations. Certainly, in rational moments, a person in an extramarital affair can see that her or his choice was a poor one. However, in the midst of pain, disappointment, a sense of failure, and the conviction that a relationship is coming apart, emotional panic takes over. Rationality temporarily disappears. If "running to someone else" in times of desperation has been a norm in the family's history, it will be a learned automatic response or inclination for the next generations as well. Such a dynamic could be taking place in any of the situations described at the beginning of this chapter. An affair, then, can be a primitive response to a feeling of desperation, loneliness, or failure. Emotionally, the person did not "know" anything else to do. This is sad, but often true.

Triangulation

The term "triangulation" in family systems theory refers to a pattern in which two people who are not handling their relationship well "triangulate" a third person to carry some of the anxiety and stress that they are not able to handle well as a twosome, or dyad. In one way, triangulation is an attempt to stabilize a troubled relationship without the partners' having to change the way they deal with each other. In other words, they are "enabled" to continue to attack, ignore, or avoid dealing with their problems by using the third person as a buffer of some kind. Some third parties cooperate unknowingly. Others do so knowingly, for reasons of their own. Still others, upon seeing what is happening, refuse to get involved.

The third party can be a child, a friend, an extended family member—even a pastor. As noted above, the function shared in common by these third parties is to keep the married partners together. A problem child keeps an otherwise alienated couple together out of their need to control or care for the child. A friend runs back and forth carrying messages of encouragement and/or gossip between an alienated couple, keeping them together by helping them avoid dealing with each other directly. An extended family member, or even several relatives, keep each party feeling too guilty to get better and too guilty to come apart. An ill-trained or poorly functioning pastor can do the same thing.

Another candidate for third party in a triangulated situation is an affair partner. Ironically for such a person, the function really being served is to keep the couple together or to create circumstances dramatic and upsetting enough to provoke more serious work on reconciliation. The affair partner is "triangulated" into the situation in a way that provides an unusual form of stability. Unfortunately, the stability often is of a kind that helps to promote avoidance of coming to terms with deeper problems. For either or both of the married partners, the affair "drains off" frustration that in a healthier relationship would lead couples to work on their difficulties. Their frustration with each other is converted into passion (anger, romantic fantasy) focused on someone else, further depleting the emotional energy that might ordinarily fuel problem-solving.

Of course, such a role is not ordinarily the conscious intent of an affair partner, but the function is served nonetheless. Hence, there are numerous stories of affair partners who are left feeling guilty and used after waiting to no avail for a divorce to make their secret relationship more "honest." Sooner—or much later—they discover themselves to have been a pawn in the unhealthy dynamics of a troubled marriage. Incidentally, the affair partner is another person in need of pastoral care. Yet he or she is often ignored or becomes the recipient of anger and condemnation from former lover, the lover's spouse, and the community at large.

The major characteristic of triangulation is that the third party takes the place of healthy communication between marital partners who do not know how to maintain or are unwilling to promote and participate in healthy communication between themselves. The "triangulee" is a substitute. A third party in the form of a professional or other caring person can be genuinely helpful to the building of bridges that eventually eliminate the need for such an intervening party. When the third party is an affair partner, the outcome is seldom redemptive.

Transference

Affairs can be triggered by special needs or even gratitude. A different kind of substitution is involved in the psychotherapeutic concept of transference. In transference, we react to a person *as if* he or she were someone or something else—usually from the past. For example, a couple in a healthy marriage may get into an argument and realize that one or both of them are more angry than the present situation warrants. If reasonably self-aware, one or both will realize that the anger is not only about the present issue but also about the fact that someone or something else frustrates or frustrated them in a similar way. In such a case, feelings from another relationship or situation are transferred into this one, compounding the intensity of the emotion.

Transference can and does appear in a variety of ways. If you have ever found yourself tearful and upset at a funeral for someone whom you did not know well, you have experienced transference. You, of course, were not grieving primarily for the person being remembered at that particular funeral. Rather, you were dealing with some grief from your past, triggered by the present funeral setting and transferred to the present. A spouse may call out, "Come here!" and you find yourself reacting with irritation. Yet you know that no hostility was intended by your wife or husband. If you think about it, however, that phrase—"come here"— may be the very one used by your father or mother when you knew you were about to be teased or embarrassed.

Feelings of love can be transferred just the same as feelings of grief and irritation. Hence, an affair is often a transference phenomenon. Most of us have been through situations in which we felt intensely attracted to someone only to wonder later where all that feeling came from. We probably had transferred unfulfilled romantic feelings from an earlier relationship onto that person and literally "saw" emotionally what we wished had been the case before. Finally the dream faded and we saw the real person before us. Only then could we evaluate the present relationship with a more realistic perspective.

Partners in both troubled and apparently healthy relationships experience transference feelings with other people. In a relatively healthy marriage, partners can recognize and acknowledge transference feelings for what they are, explore the memories, and even get in better touch with some hopes and dreams for the present marriage. In a troubled or shallow marriage, however, transference feelings may be overpowering. In the absence of healthy boundaries of commitment and self-awareness, a person may become caught up in an affair, stimulated by the secretiveness and intense emotion. Only later may it become possible to see what was going on and try to learn from the experience for the well-being of the present relationship. Unfortunately, that does not always happen.

Transference is a very real danger in a pastoral relationship. A person who is unhappy and troubled in a marriage often will experience the pastor as someone who really loves him or her in a way that no one else has or does. The pastor, in the mind of the other person, "becomes" the person to bring resolution and fulfillment to unresolved desires from the past. If he or she is not very careful, the pastor can experience powerful feelings, known as counter-transference, toward the parishioner. The regular occurrence of this phenomenon made it important to emphasize self-awareness and protection in chapter 1.

The power of transference makes it an important part of self-awareness. When it does occur, both opportunity and danger are present. A competent therapist has an extraordinary opportunity in working with someone who is experiencing transference-love for the therapist. To take advantage of the transference and become a lover to the patient is unacceptable. Equally unacceptable is letting the therapist's discomfort result in his or her rejecting the patient, thus leaving the patient with one more experience of frustration in finding resolution and self-esteem. The task of the therapist is to acknowledge and show regard for the person and the feelings that he or she has—even to offer encouragement for the capacity to love. Then the task is to help these feelings be seen as an opportunity for the client to learn how to love more fully and appropriately in healthy and significant relationships. Though it is not always found, the term "boundaries" is currently used in professional literature to describe crucial issues for a person/patient experiencing transference (see chapter 3). It is a very special gift for a patient to experience a relationship with a therapist or pastor who does *not* violate personal boundaries or take advantage of vulnerability.

Pastoral Practice

The foregoing theological and psychological discussions are intended to bring helpful perspective to a pastor attempting to care for any of several parties involved in an affair. After all, many people are affected: marital partner, affair partner, the marital partner involved in the affair, extended family, children, business associates, and friends. Any of these persons can be shaken by the breaking of covenants of fidelity, for such an experience leaves at least a tinge of distrust about all commitments. Who *can* you trust?

So, the first suggestion for pastoral practice with regard to affairs is to remember that *far more is at stake than sex.* Issues of trust remain long after physical involvements are over. Energy and attention need to be devoted to identifying the values, issues, fears, hopes, or intentions that led to the affair and will continue after it is over. In other words, do not stay hung up on the events. Look under them for the deeper issues. The only way that such a search can go on, however, is to listen first to the descriptions of the events themselves. The reader is referred again to the discussion of listening skills in chapter 3.

A further suggestion in working with people affected by affairs is to *reserve judgment* in terms of blame or fault. Because of the emotional intensity that surrounds infidelity, persons often expect a pastor to identify with their own impassioned point of view. The "betrayed" partner wants empathy with the feelings of outrage and hurt, which are real. The "unfaithful" partner wants sympathy with the sense of unhappiness or emptiness that led to his or her involvement. Those feelings are also real. Then, there is the third party, the affair partner. She or he ordinarily has a sense of empathy with the unfaithful partner, as well as concerns for her or his own well-being, and is convinced of the deeper "rightness" of their relationship, regardless of what "others may think."

Each of these persons has *real feelings*. All of those feelings can be understood, even appreciated and accepted, without the pastor "choosing up sides." Reserving judgment is not simply a matter of preserving some sort of professional neutrality. It is necessary if one is to maintain contact with the various parties involved. Once a judgment about fault is heard or seen from the pastor, the "favored" people hang on and others disappear. If that happens, the pastor loses any opportunity for pastoral guidance toward some form of reconciliation. Therefore, this delicate line must be walked carefully and sensitively.

The importance of maintaining contact and offering guidance is based on the premise that reconciliation of some kind is far preferable to further escalation of the conflict and hurt. Reconciliation, of course, is not understood here to mean only the restitution of a marriage. As noted earlier, there are circumstances in which over a longer period of time reunion could be far more damaging than separation. Rather, reconciliation here means the exploration and discovery of the means by which all parties are taken seriously and helped to find a redemptive outcome for what has taken place.

These first suggestions can be clarified further by recalling

92

the situations described early in this chapter. For example, it would be a tragic mistake for a pastor to move too quickly to cut off conversation and render a judgment on Jane for her proposed relationship with Bob. What is far more important than a sexual issue here is the grief that is bound to be present over the loss of her relationship with Herbert. Caring that is pastoral and redemptive in its intent will understand that more than sex is involved here. There should be a willingness to withhold judgment so that the grief and anger at her loss can be examined and understood more clearly *by Jane as well as by the pastor*.

Perhaps it is more acceptable to employ these two tactics with Jane than with Walter (of the second scenario), who seems at first blush just to be mean-spirited and in need of being "straightened out." But, again, presume more to be at stake than sex and withhold initial judgment. Buried in his words are also expressions of grief and disappointment. Whether true or not, Walter feels used by his wife, and he is acknowledging, though backhandedly, his need for love. Those feelings need to be explored without foreclosing the opportunity for growth and even reconciliation by assuming that Walter is a midlife crisis "on the make."

Jim, in the third scenario, is also to be admired for his decision, in his discomfort, to disclose a part of his past that seems to be a source of shame for him. An opportunity has been created by his nomination to church office, and it must be handled sensitively. There is no need for a quick decision.

These three illustrations, and my first two suggestions for pastoral practice, require a willingness on the part of pastors to set aside initial assumptions for the sake of redemptive possibilities. Of course, it is possible that Jane, Walter, and Jim all have ulterior motives, have no conscience, and are seeking to use the pastor as a tool to get what they want without regard to anyone's feelings. But that is the less likely possibility. They have come to the pastor, directly or indirectly, because they want to be understood and want to have "right relationships." Therefore, they deserve some pastoral restraint, a willingness to hold back on any expression of dismay or desire to "fix it" quickly. Such restraint is exercised for the sake of helping people who may be on a pilgrimage toward greater integrity and faithfulness. When such trust and restraint is misplaced, a pastor may feel foolish and "taken in." But the commitment to trying to care in a deeper way is worth the risk of feeling foolish.

A third suggestion for dealing with extramarital affairs is an *educational* one. Orient your pastoral care for these people in a way that *promotes self-awareness and strengthens them for making difficult choices*. The self-awareness, of course, is built on the assumption that people can become more sensitive to the forces that drive them into painful situations. The illustrations from the psychological discussion of family of origin, triangulation, and transference phenomena are concepts that may help people to understand what was (and still may be) going on that led to extramarital involvement. As awareness expands, choices will be more responsible. Some of those choices may include: confessing to an affair, ending an affair, forgiveness for an affair, willingness to go into counseling to work on a relationship, or a direct acknowledgment that a marriage is too painful and damaging to continue.

The manner in which a pastor promotes this educational process will vary widely according to the situation. It is appropriate, in the fourth and fifth scenarios, for a pastor to go to the son whose mother is concerned about the possibility of his having an affair, or to the wife whose husband is concerned, *if* there is some sort of pastoral relationship already established and *if* the concerned mother or husband is willing to tell son or wife that the concern has been discussed with you. In other words, there must be some "rite of access" that will help overcome the initial defensiveness. *Initiative* is a very important "tool" in a pastor's repertoire in dealing with extramarital affairs. It is an initiative that is best characterized by the phrase "speaking the truth in love."

Another important initiative to take in dealing with affairs is to "see to it that" the marital partners have professional help in working it through. The phrase "see to it that" is a biblical phrase that intrigues me and serves as a reminder that the pastor does not have to do everything personally. For example, the directive in Hebrews 12:15 to "see to it that no one fails to obtain the grace of God" can be interpreted as permission to a pastor to be freed from direct responsibility and to assume a more general oversight.

Working directly and frequently with the emotional intensity of an affair is a task that many pastors will not feel equipped or willing to do. In fact, general pastoral care often can be maintained more effectively if the intense work is done elsewhere. In the interests of reconciliation, whatever form it may take, the pastor can help most if he or she promotes an ongoing conversation between marital partners and with a professional counselor. In other words, if you do not feel up to it for any reason, refer. Suggestions for making referrals are given in chapter 3.

Pastoral care in dealing with extramarital affairs can be one of the most frustrating, emotionally draining, and conflict-laden experiences in ministry. Nonetheless, care of those affected by affairs is important because such deeper human needs and possibilities may become accessible if an initial tendency to be judgmental can be deterred. I hope that this chapter serves as encouragement to take on the task.

For Further Reading

A variety of perspectives are helpful in understanding the theological and psychological dynamics involved in affairs. Therefore, the recommendations here are divided into three sections: first, pastoral literature on marriage and family issues; second, psychological literature on marriage and family; third, literature on the dynamics and treatment of affairs. Titles including family are listed because much of family systems theory works with marital issues.

Pastoral Literature on Marriage and Family

Anderson, Herbert. *The Family and Pastoral Care*. Philadelphia: Fortress Press, 1984.

Biddle, Perry. *The Goodness of Marriage: A Devotional Book for Newlyweds*. Nashville: The Upper Room, 1984.

Carmody, Denise L. *Caring for Marriage: Feminist and Biblical Reflections*. Ramsey, N.J.: Paulist Press, 1985.

Fishburn, Janet. *Confronting the Idolatry of Family: A New Vision for the Household of God*. Nashville: Abingdon Press, 1991.

Mace, David R. *Love and Anger in Marriage*. Grand Rapids: Zondervan Publishing House, 1990.

Patton, John, and Brian Childs. *Christian Marriage and Family*. Nashville: Abingdon Press, 1988.

Sawyers, Lindell, ed. *Faith and Families*. Philadelphia: Geneva Press, 1986.

Thatcher, Floyd, and Harriett Thatcher. *Long Term Marriage: A Search for the Ingredients of a Lifetime Partnership*. Waco, Tex.: Word Books, 1980.

Psychological Literature on Marriage and Family

Barbach, Lonnie, and David L. Geisinger. *Going the Distance: Secrets to Lifelong Love*. New York: Doubleday, 1991.

Barbeau, Clayton. *Delivering the Male: Out of the Tough-Guy Trap and into a Better Marriage*. Minneapolis: Winston Press, 1982.

Dinkmeyer, Don C., and Jan Carlson. *Taking Time for Love: How to Stay Happily Married*. New York: Prentice-Hall, 1989.

Johnson, Catherine. *Lucky in Love: The Secrets of Happy Couples and How Their Marriages Thrive*. New York: Viking Press, 1992.

Sager, Clifford, and Bernice Hunt. *Intimate Partners: Hidden Patterns in Love Relationships*. New York: McGraw-Hill, 1979.

Scanzoni, John, et al. *The Sexual Bond: Rethinking Families and Close Relationships*. Newbury Park, Calif.: Sage Publications, 1989.

Scanzoni, Letha. *Men, Women, and Change: A Sociology of Marriage and Family*. 3d ed. New York: McGraw-Hill, 1988.

Weeks, Gerald R., ed. *Treating Couples: The Intersystem Model of the Marriage Council of Philadelphia*. New York: Brunner/Mazel, 1989.

Literature on Affairs

Brown, Emily M. *Patterns of Infidelity and Their Treatment*. New York: Brunner/Mazel, 1991.

Carnes, Patrick. *Out of the Shadows: Understanding Sexual Addiction*. Minneapolis: CompCare Publishers, 1983.

Lawson, Annette. *Adultery: An Analysis of Love and Betrayal*. New York: Basic Books, 1988.

Petersen, J. Allan. *The Myth of the Greener Grass*. Wheaton, Ill.: Tyndale House Publishers, 1983.

Pittman, Frank S. *Private Lies: Infidelity and the Betrayal of Intimacy*. New York: W. W. Norton & Co., 1990.

Saul, Leon Joseph. *Fidelity and Infidelity: And What Makes and Breaks a Marriage*. Philadelphia: J. B. Lippincott Co., 1967.

Strean, Herbert S. *The Extramarital Affair*. New York: Free Press, 1980.

6

Sexual Discrimination and Abuse

Evidence of sexual discrimination ranges from (1) the outright refusal to consider a woman (or a man) for a job because of gender to (2) the conscious or unconscious use of language to create and support an ethos that lowers the importance and worth of one gender to (3) covert and overt sexual harassment on the job or at home. Most tragic of all is the sexual abuse that takes place in the forms of incest, rape, and other physical and/or psychological cruelty. Since human ignorance, non-awareness, and cruelty sometimes seem unlimited in their manifestations, many other forms of sexual discrimination and abuse exist as well.

Public consciousness of the problem is increasing. Recent history has shown increased awareness of and willingness to acknowledge openly and confront the discrimination and abuse that has been exerted against women. Much remains to be done. Discrimination is seldom a simple and one-sided phenomenon, though the suffering of some groups (in this case, women) is usually more visible in terms of gender bias. Males also suffer and are victimized by chauvinism. We all lose. Discrimination in all its forms is wrong. This chapter will highlight several issues and suggest pastoral strategies for confronting them. We will begin the discussion with four incidents in which sexual discrimination or harassment led to, or were involved with, pastoral contacts.

Jill called her pastor shortly after her husband announced that he wanted a divorce. Although the problems in their marriage had been going on for some time, she had not expected this decision. As she talked about her fears of being alone and her need for someone who genuinely cared for her, Mark, the pastor, pulled his chair closer to her and took her hand. "Jill," he said, "don't worry. I care for you a great deal, and I am willing to be with you anytime." After that conversation, Mark called her daily and suggested more frequent visits to his office. Jill felt increasingly uncomfortable with the exorbitant amount of attention he was paying to her, but she didn't feel free to say so. After all, he was just being a good pastor, wasn't he? Then she had lunch one day with her friend Julie. When Jill began to talk of the pastoral visits from Mark, Julie rolled her eyes and said, "Don't tell me he's pulling that old 'I care for you' routine on you!"

Alice, an energetic and intelligent young lawyer, came to her pastor to talk. She had been offered a position with an old and distinguished law firm. The terms were excellent, but she knew that no woman had ever been made a partner. When she asked for some assurance of eventual consideration for partnership, the interviewing committee suggested that she not press the matter. Change was slow, they admitted, but she could trust them to work it out over time instead of "pushing it" at this early stage. "What should I do?" she asked. "I want the job, but I am being asked to trust a group of men who may want a woman in the firm for appearances but not in a position to exercise real power."

Roger, a talented professor in the local community college for fifteen years, called his pastor for an appointment. He was discouraged. In applying for a number of university positions, he had been told repeatedly that "white males" were not going to be considered seriously if women or minority candidates were available. "I feel caught," he said. "I agree with the premise that women have gotten short shrift, and I have supported many women seeking to advance. But, I'm also angry that I can't get a hearing with a search committee because I'm the wrong gender. What can I do?"

After the worship service on Sunday morning, Fred and Margaret waited until most of the other congregants had left. Then they stepped up to Joe, their pastor, at the front door. "We need to talk," said Fred. "Margaret doesn't want to come back to church anymore, because the language is offensive to her. I think she's being silly. Just tell her, Joe. All those hymns that say 'mankind' mean all of us, don't they?"

The Theological

At first glance, an appeal to the Bible for perspective on issues of gender discrimination seems to present a number of difficulties. After all, the Bible itself has much in it that is male-biased. In Old Testament law, women were treated as chattel property and thus subject to the will and power of men. Male children clearly received favor over females. And, of course, references to God use male pronouns almost exclusively. In short, it seems clear that masculinity is elevated over femininity.

The Value and Worth of Males and Females

Biblical sources have been used to support an array of practices bestowing power and privilege on males and withholding it from females. The Roman Catholic practice of ordaining only men as priests is one of the most enduring reminders of such practices, but blatant and subtle vestiges are also found throughout Christendom. As a result, many women have been discouraged and angry with the church as they seek to overcome the cultural prejudice that has worked against them. Why remain, they ask, in a church that regularly responds to them as does the larger culture—with unequal pay for equal work, with "old-boy networks" that exclude them from real participation in major decisions, and with harassment from male clergy and lay persons alike.

But wait! That's not the whole picture. Continuing biblical and theological studies show that much of our understanding of the Bible has been shaped by generations of translators and interpreters who themselves were distorted in their perspective because of male-dominated forms of thinking and perceiving. A few examples will be discussed here, and suggestions for further reading are offered at the end of the chapter.

In the creation accounts of the book of Genesis, there is a remarkable description of "the man" and "the woman" and the relationship that God intended for them. The story is particularly striking because it seems to contradict the lowered status of women in the culture at the time when the accounts were written.

Two passages will illustrate. The first is in Genesis 1:27, where humankind is described as created in God's image—male and female. *Both* reflect the image of God, without elevation of one over the other. The second is in Genesis 2:18, as the search begins for a helper who will be a genuine partner to the man, because God sees it to be "not good" that the man is alone. Though "helper" has often been construed to mean a kind of servant, the fact that the helper specifically is to be a genuine partner brings a note of equality to the intended relationship. This intended equality becomes more clear in the "search process" that followed. Many creatures are deemed *not* to have the capacity to be genuine partners, so the woman is created and is declared to meet the requirement. Here, embedded in the midst of a culture that diminished women, stands a story that declares God's opposing view. Women are beings who, with men, reflect the image of God and are to stand in full partnership with them. Such a radical view can be an impressive argument for the inspiration of scripture—it is surely not a mere reflection of the culture in which it was written.

Of course, the message of female value is one that is then contradicted many times in subsequent scripture, but this beginning stance in the Genesis "orders of creation" reappears time and time again. The culmination is found in Jesus' attitudes as he confirms the original creation intentions by valuing, respecting, and associating with women. While Jesus chose men to be disciples, it must also be noted that those male disciples frequently just "didn't get it" with regard to Jesus' message. In fact, they often are shown to be foolish in their competition for status and power. Consistently, a group of women, many of whom are not even named, do "get it" and stand faithfully by Jesus when the men are running for cover.

While we cannot undertake here a detailed and comprehensive study of the issue of male and female worth in scripture, these few observations are consistent with more extensively developed views. The sum of them is that women and men are created to be equal partners in service to God. As such, they are called to respect each other and to stand together over against actions and beliefs that depreciate either women or men, individually or collectively.

Such theological affirmations are important fodder for pastoral conversations such as those identified earlier in this chapter. Fred and Margaret, in their all-too-typical conversation at the front door of the church after worship, raise the issue of language. The concerns expressed by each of them (even though Margaret hasn't spoken yet!) call for careful, sensitive, and candid care from Joe, the pastor. Care here must include the pastor's own self-awareness, because the situation serves as a reminder of the power of his language to shape perceptions.

The Role of Finitude and Sin

This next theological reminder returns us to the discussion of finitude and sin begun in chapter 2. Much misunderstanding that results in outright discrimination or abuse grows out of our limited capacity to understand and value differences. The creation passages discussed above note that God created male and female to reflect the image of God. The widely diverse characteristics and capacities of male and female are indicative of the vastness and diversity of God's own being. In fact, part of the problem of male/female relationships lies in the reality that genders can be so different that they do not understand each other. Yet, at the same time, there are enough similarities that women and men are drawn to each other. Those characteristics give testimony to the wideness of God's being—so wide that they seem unrelated. At the same time, they give testimony to the coherence and unity of God's being. The parts, our gender characteristics, as magnets, seem to both attract and repel.

In their search for security and relief from tension, people are often prone to ignore their limitations and attempt to encourage sameness: "Be like me so that I won't have to struggle with you." When encouragement fails, desperation may take over and attempt to guarantee security by diminishing, if not outright destroying, those who are different from themselves. Human history is filled with examples. It is in such a response to finitude that humans participate, consciously or unconsciously, in sin. Anxiety is indeed a breeding ground for sin.

The Bible not only reflects God's intentions, but it also provides us with gutsy and dismaying "case studies" of the sin committed in human searches for "unnatural" security and autonomy. From this perspective, sexual discrimination must be understood as being something other than sexual at its base. Gender, and the differences implied in it, becomes one of many platforms on which human beings seek to elevate themselves. When discrimination occurs, the interaction is no longer sexual; rather, it is indicative of a struggle for power.

Mark, the pastor in our earlier illustration, affirms himself by flaunting his power to "move in" with relative freedom on someone, in this case, a woman. In a similar but more "civilized" way, Alice, the lawyer, is asked to remain weak and let "the men" take care of her and the firm. Roger, the professor in search of a new job, finds himself the victim of the history of male chauvinism. He now suffers the same unjustified discrimination that women have faced for years. Fred, the loyal church member, in his lack of understanding of what it is like to feel ignored by the language of the worship service, wants Margaret to just "understand" that she is included—so that he will not have to be uncomfortably challenged to hear scripture in a new way.

The Psychological and the Physical

Close linkage exists between our theological affirmations and psychological studies that inform us about "what is going on" with us human beings. Psychology offers us a variety of ways to classify and understand further what underlies the ways in which human beings treat each other with both acceptance and disdain, both knowingly and unknowingly.

The struggle for power is an age-old issue, as noted in our theological comments above. One of a number of psychological perspectives revolves around *gender differences*. From both psychological observation and biological exploration, as noted in chapter 2, there do seem to be some "typical" differences beyond the anatomical ones between males and females. One of them has to do with aggression. Males, typically, are more aggressive than females. Such patterns have been observed, for example, in studies of children's play and studies of the expression of anger.

Males, particularly when they are unsure or unaware of what is going on and what is at stake for them, frequently use physical strength to exercise control and get what they want. Their actions in the sexual realm can range from rape to physical abuse to threats of physical harm to harassment and ridicule—all exercised as a way of "overpowering" another person (other men as well as women). What might be described as "just having a little fun" or as "special affection" is often a clear disrespect for and willingness to take advantage of "weakness," however defined, in the other person. It can even serve as a means to deny or ignore one's own anxieties by "putting down" or exercising control over the vulnerabilities of another.

Other common, though not universal, differences between the genders that often lead to discrimination, or at least misunderstanding, are the male inclination to "fix" problems, in contrast to a female inclination to be empathetic in "understanding" problems. Sometimes that "fixing" takes the form of physical control, insensitive to the effects of that exercise of power on another person's feelings.

Men tend to be more oriented toward gaining and exchanging *information*, while women are more likely to build rapport around common *feelings*. This, too, contributes to difficulties illustrated by Martha and Christopher in chapter 4, where he perceived Martha's attempts to "inform" as attempts to take control by knowing more than he. For some men, such a perception becomes a justification for physical violence.

A further psychological perspective that contributes to an understanding (but not acceptance) of discriminatory and even abusive treatment revolves around the concept of *narcissism*. A number of theories exist as to the causes of narcissism, but it is lived out in a self-preoccupation that genuinely does not understand or care to understand another person's point of view. The lifestyle of such a person might be characterized as "I want what I want when I want it." Out of arrogance or psychological myopia, the narcissist runs roughshod over other people's feelings, concerns, and even rights. Hence, others are used—physically, economically, socially. A spouse, whether male or female, is seen as there to "serve." To use our theological language, the finitude of being able to see only the needs of the self leads to the sin of seeing others as only to be used for one's own desires. Strict and forthright controls often have to be set for such a person.

Finally, another powerful psychological lens is to be found in the framework of one's *family of origin*. There are indeed families who manifest an ethic of discrimination and exaggerated control. People are, literally, "trained" to be discriminatory by their families of origin. In many traditional families, women have *always* been expected to serve the men. Men have *always* been expected to earn the living. Women have always been taught that they are to remain quiet after being beaten, or to turn their money over to the man. Men have always been taught to deny feelings and appear strong. When people have been raised with such norms as their only frame of reference, it is not a surprise to us that they treat people outside of the family in the same way. Families of origin are powerful forces. Not only do they teach their members how to "be," but they also teach their members what to see and not see, what to think and not think, what to feel and not feel. The sad result is a seriously dysfunctional family in which sexual discrimination and harassment are perceived as "normal." Equality and fairness are seen as weak and ineffective.

Dynamics of power, gender differences, narcissism, and family-of-origin issues are only some of the perspectives that help us to understand acts of blatant physical, psychological, economic, and social harm to others because of gender. One of our pastoral responsibilities is to attempt to lessen the damage, or at least provide eyes to see and ears to hear.

Pastoral Practice

The tasks of pastoral care broaden when issues of sexual discrimination and abuse are faced. There is still the responsibility to hear and provide information. However, there is often an added responsibility to set limits and even provide protection. Because of the variety of ways in which sexual discrimination may occur, it is important to develop an orientation that is a bit more investigative.

The importance of *listening* cannot be overemphasized here. Because of the high profile that issues of abuse and harassment are receiving in our society, some people will use those words to gain an immediate level of sympathy. Pastors have to develop gifts of discernment to distinguish between those who falsely allege sexual discrimination, those who are genuine in their complaint or fear, and those who are too fearful to acknowledge the hurt that they have suffered. As noted in chapter 3, it is important for a pastor to hear the whole story with minimal interruptions. The listening should be full, attending not only to the words of the story but to the nonverbal signals as well. Note the places that do not seem to quite fit or the places in which something seems to be left out or passed over quickly. Then, when the story has been told and the time is right, go back in a spirit of gentle, but persistent, inquiry to get the fuller story.

There will be times, illustrated by several of our earlier pastoral situations, in which *education* will be needed. In the case of Fred and Margaret, a similar strategy can be adopted. The pastor needs to hear both of them, but it is even more important that they hear each other. Fred needs to know of Margaret's feelings of being invisible because of the absence of references to females in worship. Margaret needs to know of Fred's fears and anxiety about changing the language of worship. For both of them the issue is more than a matter of specific words. The words provide access to far deeper and more crucial matters about each person's self-regard and their perceptions of how they are regarded by each other and by God. It is probable that neither of these two people have told each other directly and specifically of such things as regard or self-esteem. Consequently, they did not really *know*. For Fred and Margaret to *learn* these things about each other is educational in the fullest sense of the word, preparing them for fuller intimacy.

In addition to listening and education there may well be needs for the provision of *structure*, since we have said one of the functions of pastoral care is to provide a sense of safe harbor in the midst of experienced threat or chaos.

The forms of structure may vary widely. In the case of Alice, the lawyer, a listening structure is provided simply by her being able to talk about her anxiety and anger about the employment opportunity she seeks. However, an additional form of structure could be an introduction to another attorney who would serve as advocate and advisor in handling her ongoing conversation with the law firm. A community of faith usually has a number of professional people who can be called upon for their expertise in particular situations. Having a professional consultation resource group in place is a valuable form of pastoral care. Furthermore, it puts flesh on the concept of the priesthood of all believers. In that wider priesthood are people who know more than we and who can be helpful in the decision-making process in which Alice finds herself. That same sort of opportunity could be made available to Roger, the professor, as he wrestles with his sense of being discriminated against in the academic world.

Every pastor and every congregation needs to provide pastoral care through the assurance of *protection* from harassment and/or abuse within the church itself. Several references have been made in this book to the tragic cases in which pastors and

107

other professional persons have taken sexual advantage of parishioners or clients. Our particular illustration in this chapter is that of Mark, the pastor. A formal process for dealing with sexual harassment and the willingness to implement the process both needed to be in place. Such a mechanism could have been used to set limits for Mark swiftly and without apology. The sad fact is that in many such cases churches or other professional groups have been hesitant to set limits on the offending party. Consequently, many people, primarily women, have been harmed and had neither recourse nor support from the church or denomination to which the offending pastor or church employee was related.

The protection recommended here is a formal policy to be employed in cases of alleged or suspected sexual misconduct. It is very important that the mechanisms for implementing the policy be in place and be generally known. Several purposes are served by this. First, public notice is given that the church takes sexuality and our human vulnerability seriously. Second, gender is affirmed as a sacred dimension of who we are as human beings. Furthermore, our belief in the richness that God intends for relationships is openly affirmed. Third, a policy on sexual misconduct serves warning on those who are tempted to take advantage of the vulnerability of others. It also gives courage to those who fear that their hurt will not be taken seriously. Fourth, the process of designing such a policy serves in itself as a major educational opportunity for a congregation.

Policy formulation may not seem like pastoral care, but, increasingly, it is. The need for such policies grows out of innumerable occasions in which pastors have heard tragic stories in the privacy of their studies. Rape, incest, and spouse abuse are increasingly evident in our world. Pastors have the "data" to persuade congregations of the immensity of the problem and can walk the delicate balance between continuing to hear the private hurts and becoming advocates for those who are not ready or able to "go public."

A Special Note on Care for the Sexually Abused

Much of this chapter has concentrated on the less dramatic, but nonetheless hurtful, incidents of discrimination and harassment that occur everyday. We would like to wish it were not so, but research increasingly confirms, and forces us to acknowledge, that sexual abuse is far more common in our world and in our culture than we ever thought. Sexual abuse here means incest, rape, and/or any other form of physical and psychological seduction of a person for one's own satisfaction without adequate regard for the full and knowing consent of, or for the impact on, that person. In other words, abuse is the unmitigated exercise of power to *use* another person for one's own pleasure or satisfaction. Again, some illustrative cases will be used to illuminate the discussion.

—College campuses have begun (in some cases, sadly, it has been necessary to force them to do so) to introduce protective and educational programs to combat the frequent incidence of rape, date rape, and acquaintance rape. Counseling services are deluged with the problem at the start of the academic year when new, "innocent" first-year students have arrived on campus.

—In September 1991, at a Las Vegas naval gathering, partying Navy and Marine aviators formed a "gauntlet" in the third-floor hallway of their hotel and jeered and pawed at the breasts and buttocks of any woman who was unfortunate enough to walk by. An official inquiry was launched only after persistent publicity and formal charges, and many of the pilots who had known of the harassment refused to cooperate with the investigation. Following the announcement of a suspension of all naval promotions until completion of the investigation, a naval officer went to his chaplain to talk. He could not understand, he said, why the government was making such a "big deal" out of this. Sure, "maybe it got a bit out of hand, but the guys were just having a little fun."

—A pastor received a call from a concerned parishioner and mother of an eighteen-month-old child. "I don't know what to make of this," she said, "but the last two times that we have left

Susan with one of our babysitters, she has asked us not to leave. Later, when I asked her why, she said, 'Because he always licks my bottom after I take my bath.'"

Cases of spouse-beating have received much attention in the media in recent years, and many public figures have made statements about the abuse they have watched or experienced during their own childhoods. Pastors receive pressure both to give attention to this in parish educational programs and not to talk about it because it is so distasteful. Nonetheless, regardless of any public and/or programmatic steps taken or not taken in a congregation, private and secretive reports that call for attention are likely to be made to a parish pastor.

References have been made here and earlier in this chapter to blatant behavior that results in rape, spouse abuse, and incest. These acts are not sexual; they are expressions of rage and unmitigated exercises of power.

Fortunately, instead of hiding behind easy phrases like "not interfering with family life or the private relationships of men and women," many segments of our culture are becoming more willing to acknowledge these acts for what they are. Pastors increasingly will be in the position of "hearing first" about such acts. On those occasions, a pastor holds responsibility both to the offender and to the victim.

For the offender, the pastor's responsibility is to take whatever action is necessary to set strict limits on the person's interaction with the victim. If a minister is not careful, pastoral care's traditional emphasis on gentle and listening support may be useful to an offender. But understanding is not enough. The offender must be stopped! In most states, because pastors have a legal responsibility to report abusive acts and patterns, it is important for clergy to know the law in their state. Furthermore, pastors have a moral obligation to state candidly and forthrightly to the offender that the offender's actions are wrong and unacceptable. Whatever boundaries the pastor can set should be put in place immediately. To do so is not only to protect the victim, it also ultimately benefits the offender.

Along with the responsibility to stop and prevent harm, the pastor has a responsibility to attempt to find appropriate treatment for the offender. Many abusers' groups exist now, and offenders should be encouraged to join one even if a legal requirement to do so is not imposed. In addition to seeing that professional therapeutic help is obtained for the offender, the pastor should maintain contact with him or her if possible. Angered and even repulsed as we may be at such acts, the origins of this kind of behavior often cry out for care.

Of course, education toward understanding of self and others is still important both for the offender and those who sympathize with offenders. For example, the young aviator who complains of having his "fun" taken too seriously needs to learn some things—theologically and psychologically—about taking other human beings seriously. Furthermore, he needs to hear clearly the effects of his perceived playfulness. Education in this case might even take the form of arranging a conversation for him with a woman who has been harassed, abused, or even raped. Such a pastoral move would be a response designed to take both the aviator and women seriously, giving both an opportunity to have consciousness and a sense of morality raised in a number of ways.

Pastoral care *for the victim* of abuse, rape, and/or incest is crucial and delicate. These persons will be "in recovery" for a long time, if not a lifetime. Their age, the circumstances surrounding the abuse, and the victim's previous relationship to the offender all shape the hurt and lingering pain. One understandable characteristic shared by many abused persons is suspicion of anyone who offers care. After all, the source of their distress may well have been a person who claimed to be nurturing. The victim is in recovery because of his or her previous vulnerability. Care invites vulnerability, which is the very thing they do not want to make available again.

So, pastoral care of the recovering victim of sexual abuse must be of a special quality. All the boundaries discussed in chapter 3—space and place, time, language, touch (especially), and awareness and careful monitoring of the pastor's own feelings—

must be provided and made absolutely clear. Particular understanding must be developed and respect shown for the victim's
necessarily long, slow redevelopment of trust and the ability to
live with a sense of relative safety.

Specifically, awareness of the grief process will be of help.
Although more than grief is going on, a profound awareness of
some loss—perhaps of innocence, of a feeling of relative safety, of
belief in one's ability to be a good judge of other people, of a variety of hopes and dreams—is present much of the time. For example, the mother of the child molested by the babysitter
struggled with guilt and the loss of confidence in leaving her
child with anyone. All pastors need to take time to read and study
more deeply about this aspect of recovery. A surprising number
of people are going through it—indeed, you may be going
through it yourself!

Finally, pastors have a responsibility to extend care to *congregations and the wider community* by making sexual harassment, misconduct, and abuse "speakable." For too long abusers have been
able to continue their harm to others because people looked the
other way. Motivations for avoiding confrontation—embarrassment, discomfort, fear of retaliation, the mistaken belief that
abuse is usually the victim's fault, the awareness that such confrontation will be a long and arduous process—vary widely. Whatever they are, however, those reservations must be overcome out
of the moral obligation to care for and protect victims. Much can
be done to advance justice and care for both offender and abused
by "giving permission" to congregations and individuals to ad-
dress these issues of sexual misconduct and abuse. For the pastor
to speak of them in both personal conversation and in public ser-
mons and prayers does much to build a community of caring.

For Further Reading

A remarkable amount of literature has appeared recently in
religious as well as more general publications on harassment and
abuse. The Mennonite Central Committee in Akron, Pennsyl-

vania, has done a particularly helpful job in preparing packets and information on the subject. I am grateful that their materials have pointed me to a number of books, tapes, and training literature of which I had not been aware.

The first list, focused on abuse within the church, contains some of the titles given at the end of chapter 3.

Baker, Don. *Beyond Forgiveness: The Healing Touch of Church Discipline*. Portland, Ore.: Multnomah Press, 1984.

Brown, Joanne Carlson, and Carole R. Bohn, eds. *Christianity, Patriarchy, and Abuse: A Feminist Critique*. New York: Pilgrim Press, 1989.

Fortune, Marie M. *Is Nothing Sacred? When Sex Invades the Pastoral Relationship*. San Francisco: Harper & Row, 1989.

———. *Keeping the Faith: Questions and Answers for the Abused Woman*. San Francisco: Harper & Row, 1989.

———. *Sexual Violence: The Unmentionable Sin*. New York: Pilgrim Press, 1983.

Glas, Maxine, and Jeanne Stevenson-Moessner. *Women in Travail and Transition: A New Pastoral Care*. Philadelphia: Fortress Press, 1991.

Horton, Anne L., and Judith A. Williamson, eds. *Abuse and Religion: When Praying Isn't Enough*. Lexington, Mass.: Lexington Books, 1988.

Hyde, Margaret O. *Sexual Abuse—Let's Talk About It*. Rev. ed. Philadelphia: Westminster Press, 1987.

Lebacqz, Karen. *Professional Ethics—Power and Paradox*. Nashville: Abingdon Press, 1985.

Lebacqz, Karen, and Ronald G. Barton. *Sex in the Parish*. Louisville, Ky.: Westminster/John Knox Press, 1991.

Leehan, James. *Pastoral Care for Survivors of Family Abuse*. Louisville, Ky.: Westminster/John Knox Press, 1989.

McDonald, John D. *One More Sunday*. New York: Ballantine Books, 1984.

Muck, Terry C., ed. *Sins of the Body*. Waco, Tex.: Word Books, 1989.

Pellauer, Mary D., Barbara Chester, and Jane A. Boyajian, eds. *Sexual Assault and Abuse: A Handbook for Clergy and Religious Professionals*. San Francisco: Harper & Row, 1987.

Rediger, G. Lloyd. *Ministry and Sexuality: Cases, Counseling, and Care*. Philadelphia: Fortress Press, 1990.

Sexual Abuse: The Church's Responsibility for the Safety of Children, Youth, and Vulnerable Adults. Washington Association of Churches, 4759 15th Avenue, N.E., Seattle, WA, 98105.

More general works in professional and popular literature include:

Bass, Ellen, and Laura Davis. *The Courage to Heal: A Guide for Women Survivors of Child Sexual Abuse*. San Franciso: Harper & Row, 1988.

Blume, E. Sue. *Secret Survivors: Uncovering Incest and Its Aftereffects in Women*. New York: John Wiley and Sons, 1990.

Boston Women's Health Book Collective. *The New Our Bodies, Ourselves*. Boston: Simon & Schuster, 1985.

Davis, Laura. *The Courage to Heal Workbook: For Women and Men Survivors of Child Sexual Abuse*. San Francisco: Harper-San Francisco, 1990.

Groth, N., with J. Birnbaum. *Men Who Rape*. New York: Plenum Press, 1979.

Maltz, Wendy. *The Sexual Healing Journey: A Guide for Survivors of Sexual Abuse*. New York: HarperCollins, 1991.

Russel, Diane. *Sexual Exploitation: Rape, Child Sexual Abuse, and Workplace Harassment*. Newbury Park, Calif.: Sage Publications, 1984.

Walker, M., and S. Brody, eds. *Sexual Assault: The Victim and the Rapist*. Lexington, Mass.: Lexington Books, 1976.

7
Sexuality and Adolescence

While the other issues discussed thus far stimulate a great deal of concern, probably those pertaining to adolescence provoke the most open and frequent comment. Most congregations have frequent formal and informal discussions about "what to do with our youth." Congregations and denominations have funded multiple studies and proposals about youth ministry. This concern stems from, among other things, lack of participation on the part of youth in the life of the church, fears about the use of drugs, and this book's particular concern—sex. Again, we will begin with some pastoral incidents.

A pastor, freshly arrived at his new place of service, was unpacking his books at the church. It was late in the afternoon and he was sweaty and tired, so he was not pleased to hear a soft knock at the door. "Are you the new preacher?" asked a young man, whom the pastor later found to be eighteen years old. "Yes," was the reply. "Well, I need some help," said the young man. "My girl friend was supposed to get her period this morning, and she didn't—so I guess that means we need to get married."

Martha called her pastor early one morning. "Mary is pregnant," she said. "She wants an abortion and needs my consent. I agree that she is too young for a child, but I think her father will insist on her having the baby. Can you go with us to the abortion clinic today? I need someone to be with me."

"When is the church going to take a stand, preacher?" Jason, a father himself, was furious. "I know those kids are drinking and having sex every weekend. Someone has to make sure that they stop it, and we're counting on you to stand up for what's right."

"I know that Christians aren't supposed to have sex before they're married," said Marcia, sitting in her pastor's study, "and I know that sex is dangerous, with AIDS and everything. But I love him, and we plan to marry after we finish high school and college and get good jobs. Isn't sex really for the one you love, to express how much you love each other? Isn't that what God really intended?"

The Theological

An excursion into scripture and the theological tradition for clear advice on sexuality and adolescence can be a frustrating enterprise. There are no obvious texts or early church fathers (or mothers) to whom to appeal. In fact, adolescence as a concept is a relatively modern "invention."

What can be found are stories that confirm for us the impulsiveness and impatience that are so often characterized as the "nature" of teenagers. Cain kills his brother, Abel (Gen. 4); brothers Jacob and Esau have their own conflicts (Gen. 25:25ff.); Joseph and his brothers go through jealousies over who is their father's favorite (Gen. 37ff.); David and Jonathan pursue their friendship in spite of Saul's prohibitions (1 Sam. 18ff.); Ruth faithfully cares for Naomi (Ruth 1). Those are some of the Old Testament stories, mostly about males and mostly showing the drive of young males to get what they want when they want it. Stories of young females are more rare and frequently model patience and willingness to wait. These anecdotes are caricatures, certainly, but they do point to some of the differences between males and females that we have discussed already.

New Testament stories about adolescents are even more rare, though Paul's gentle leading and caring for his young follower, Timothy (see Phil. 2:19–22), may offer some clues about the nature of caring relationships with those younger than us. Of course, it is speculation to call any of these people adolescents, since there are few concrete references to their ages in these stories.

Several things can be noted, however. First, the Bible itself gives abundant documentation of the fact that we human beings cannot fully control or assure the direction of our children's lives, or those of anyone else's children, for that matter. The encouragement, if not outright command, that is urged upon Christians is to be models for those younger than us. Furthermore, we are called to encourage in teenagers a wider awareness of and restraint from activities that threaten harm to the self or to another. There are both encouragements and warnings about the roles of parents. Warnings include the damage that can be done to children through mistakes and poor modeling (see the discussion in chapter 5 on family-of-origin issues).

In other words, scripture continues to offer a marvelous balance between visions of things to be hoped for and texts that drive home the reality that human life is beyond our full control. To live in that balance, "between the times," requires an understanding of human beings as stewards, rather than owners, of the creation in which we live and of the lives that are entrusted to us. Christians are called to give testimony to that belief, which has particular implications for our relationships with children and adolescents for whom we are called to be caring listeners and supporters as we encourage them toward maturity.

The Physiological and Psychological

Biology and psychology have studied the anatomy and the psyche carefully over the years. They offer a number of specific facts that we can blend with the commitments to which we have referred in the theological section.

First, it is important to remember that dramatic bodily and psychic changes are taking place during adolescence. For most teenagers, appearances really can be deceiving. They *look* adult, but they are far from it both inside and outside.

The physiological changes, which include the growth of body hair, the onset of menstruation and growth of breasts for girls, and a range of other things familiar to any who have already been through it, engender both wonderment and lack of control concerning the physical self. And just as the boy or girl begins to puzzle over these changes, there is also a surge of hormonal activity that prompts more physical changes that leave the young person feeling even more out of control. Nocturnal emissions, vaginal moistness, erections—all are embarrassing, sometimes unexplainable, and, perhaps most important and scariest of all, uncontrollable. Frustration, impatience, and sexual urges accompany all these changes. Most confusing of all, sometimes those urges are indistinguishable from other urges. Youth workers can relate many a tale about the confusion expressed by young adolescents who are not sure whether the excitement they feel holding hands with a boyfriend or girlfriend at church camp is sexual arousal or a call to the ministry!

Writers on adolescence tend to agree that the main psychological issue during this period can be summed up in the word *identity*. Definitions of what that means will vary, of course; but most people agree that the adolescent's search is on for "what makes me who I am." It is a time of exploration and experimentation, and it is an important search. Erik Erikson characterizes this developmental period in dialectical terms, as a phase of struggle between identity and diffusion—a battle between having a sense of focus and feeling scattered, out of control.

Other writers have pointed to several areas in which this struggle and experimentation with identity go on. An example is *faithfulness*. What does it mean to be faithful and dependable and predictable? What does being faithful to something or someone do to help, hurt, cause trouble? What does it mean to be unfaithful, to break promises, to be "different"? The exploration of all this uncertainty by an adolescent is rarely conscious and conceptual, especially in the early stages, though it certainly can be. However, consciously or not, a massive "scan" of the self and the world is going on. The results of this "study" greatly affect shaping the self, gaining a sense of focus, and setting patterns for future relationships, commitments, and self-esteem.

The behavior of the adolescent, of course, is shaped by these forces and issues being experienced and explored within the self.

Because of the powerful accompanying emotions, there are a variety of ways teenagers will respond to overt attempts to guide and direct their behavior. As is characteristic of this developmental stage, the responses and reactions tend to be extreme. Some young people are excessively compliant and submissive, ready to do anything anyone tells them. Others are guaranteed to do just the opposite of what they are told. And, of course, there are all sorts of gradations in between.

What seems to be most important for the well-being of teenagers during this time of growth and change is the presence of a stable, dependable, and faithful environment to provide care and protection. Attempts to over-control may be met with compliance or rebellion. However, the adolescent's *reaction* should not be the determinant for action. To allow that would be to offer reactivity as a response to reactivity. Rather, the responsibility of adults is to maintain a mature commitment to the provision of that stable environment. The boundaries provide a contained testing ground for the young person's search for identity. If the boundaries are undependable, then the adolescent is thrown into further fears about the absence of control. Just when he or she feels undependable and changing, there appears to be nothing *outside* of himself or herself that is dependable and lasting.

Now, consider all of these characteristics of the adolescent in relationship to sex. Sexual beings are very much influenced by their bodies. The bodies of adolescents are changing, so one of their identity questions revolves around the question "What effect does my body have on my worth and value in the eyes of others—most important, in the eyes of my peers?" Consequently, major experimentation with one's body goes on, privately and in relation to others: body-building, using makeup, touching, and, of course, experimenting with physical intimacy. Voluminous amounts of energy and emotional intensity go into worrying about one's body and how it is regarded by others. One of the accompanying questions often is, "Do you have to admire or have access to my body in order to like (or love) me?"

Yet there is more to the matter than just these questions of regard or worth. It is also true that bodies can be a source of good feelings. In worry and anxiety, a very human response is to seek pleasure as a means of escaping the discomfort. Sex during adolescence (and, for that matter, in adulthood) is often "used" for that very thing. The need for relief from painful anxiety can often overrule other beliefs or scruples about what is right and acceptable. In just such circumstances lie the grounds for later feelings of guilt and/or addiction. Patterns are being set during these experiments of adolescence.

Earlier reference has been made to issues of control. In some ways, adolescence is a repeat performance of the experimental behavior that occurs around the age of two. Here, too, limits are being tested. But boundaries seem to be far more easy to establish and maintain with a two-year-old than with a teenager. With the adolescent, physical restraint is not needed so much as the provision of "safe places" to talk, to wonder, to confess, and to plan. All of this is to say that since control of the adolescent is not possible, it is far more important to provide a context within which control can be established *by* the teenager.

Pastors often occupy a position, if they will use it, of enough emotional distance from daily life with any particular teenager to provide such a safe place. It is also true that clergy can offer a valuable ministry to parents, who also need a place to regain perspective as they struggle to find a balance between over-controlling and under-controlling.

Pastoral Practice

In keeping with what has been said thus far, it is important to begin again with a word of comfort and encouragement for both parents and pastors. *We cannot fully control the behavior of teenagers.* There may have been a simpler day when that was possible, but I doubt it. A frequent comment made by teenagers when asked about strictures placed on them by parents or society is, "If we want to (drink, have sex, drive fast), we can find a way." It is true. That reality must be admitted by all adults. If not realized from the first, adults may well take extreme actions that result in later feelings of responsibility for *driving* young people into more extreme behavior than they might have undertaken otherwise. That is certainly true when dealing with sexual behavior. Furthermore, if pastors make it evident that they accept this reality when talking with an adolescent, the normal resistance they feel about discussing intimate material is likely to be reduced. The young person will be relieved to know that it will not be necessary to get into a battle over who is in control of her or his life.

Another important principle in pastoral care for youth and their families is to *find ways to be around teenagers in the church* with some regularity. That does not mean that the pastor should take over the youth program. Youth ministry is often looked at as a job for beginning pastors and something to be given up, usually by choice, later in one's pastoral career. However, if young people are to know that there is a "safe place" for them to talk, pastors need to at least "show up" at their events with some frequency. Their appearance tells young people something about pastoral interest and availability.

More specifically, pastors should *find ways to make sex and sexuality* speakable around teenagers. Give evidence of comfort with and a willingness to engage in talk about sex spontaneously and without embarrassment. In the best of all possible worlds, of course, there will be sex education programs provided by the church—even before the teenage years. But if such education has not been a part of the history of a particular congregation, youth need to know that their pastor is not uncomfortable with the topic.

Enabling the pastor to experience such comfort was one of the goals of the first chapter of this book. To speak comfortably and positively about sex in the presence of teenagers teaches them a number of things: that sex is a normal and important part of who we are as creatures made in the image of God; that sex has a proper place and role in our lives as Christians; and that sex is something that can be talked about safely any time, any place, including the privacy of the pastor's office.

If these principles are carried out reasonably well, it is fairly certain that sooner or later an adolescent, troubled about sex for any of a number of reasons, will ask for some time to talk. When those moments come, the suggestions for context given in chapter 3 are once again very important, as are the following principles, which apply to teenagers in particular.

Do not immediately get caught up in approval or disapproval of any behavior that is described. *Listen for the deeper issues that led this person to talk* about the behavior. Because of the immense sensitivity that adolescents have to approval or disapproval, they are listening very carefully for any indication of judgment. In the face of immediate judgment unaccompanied by understanding, many will leave, psychologically if not physically. It is far more important at the outset to show interest in and understanding of the feelings that are at stake in the young person's revealing what is going on or being contemplated. Only if this level of rapport can be established can *they* eventually listen. Anxiety is not conducive to good hearing.

Here again, self-awareness and comfort with the subject are something a sensitive pastor should have worked out in advance of any conversations such as this. If that homework has been done, the minister can focus on helping to reduce the anxiety of the other person instead of having to struggle primarily with his or her own.

Help the person to distinguish between feelings and actions. One of the most difficult things for human beings to do is learn that feelings can be separated from actions or choices. People are often trapped by the conviction that to feel something means that they must do something. For example, to feel "turned on" sexually no more means that someone *must* have intercourse than to feel angry means that a person must hit someone. Teenagers, as do all human beings, often have to be reminded of the choices that are really available to them.

Marcia, from our vignettes at the beginning of the chapter, may see that there are choices that she can make about whether to have intercourse with her boyfriend if her feelings for him are understood. The young man visiting the new pastor also needs help here. He has obviously already taken action, but the results of those feelings and actions still leave him with choices. Marriage is not a settled matter—but it will be if the pastor jumps right in with a recommendation or registers disapproval.

In seeking to understand the deeper issues and separation between feelings and actions, pastors need to be *listening and watching for educational opportunities*. There is always room for education, if helpfully offered. The young man who is convinced that his girlfriend is pregnant needs some lessons on biology and the menstrual cycle. Martha, who is about to head for the abortion clinic with her daughter, has a number of things that she and her daughter both need to know—and it is to be hoped that if the pastor does not help, the clinic will. The adamant father who wants teenage behavior "stopped" has a great deal to learn about working with youth. He, too, however, will only be able to learn if the fears that underlie his anger are first understood. Sex education has already been mentioned. Much anxiety takes place around sex because of things not known, especially with teenagers. In light of what *is* known about sexually transmitted diseases, particularly HIV and AIDS, an alert pastor who sees likelihood or actuality of sexual behavior among teenagers will take steps to make sure that teenagers know about safe sex.

A major gift that a pastor can bring to any teenager struggling with issues of sex is *carefully timed and sensitively articulated honesty*. When trust has been established, when verbal or nonverbal assurance has been given that power plays will not be attempted, when the pastor's regard for the young person is evident, virtually anything can be said. But none of it can helpfully be said and heard if the prior conditions have not been established.

Above all, in dealing with teenagers and sexual matters, look for opportunities to *affirm the goodness of sexuality and the context in which it is intended to be exercised*. The church has too long carried the burden of being seen as an institution that views sex as "dirty." Adolescents, for the most part, carry that view—or at least the view that people of the church get too "uptight" about sex. If sex can simply be treated as one more of the many issues that call for reflection and planning and struggle in the search for richness in life, then much will have been contributed to the growth of young people. With a rich and wholesome understanding of sex and the fact that human beings are sexual beings, the message to adolescents can be that the church is not so much uptight about sex as its people are convinced of the special place that sex holds in our being and in our lives. If anything, then, the church's concern about sex grows out of a desire to help those still growing in the faith to see it as a special dimension of who they are and to treat it with appropriate reverence in order to enjoy it most fully.

These recommendations may sound "liberal" to some. However, I view them not so much as permissive as realistic in light of who we are as human beings. Some of the most damaging effects of sex in the lives of youth grow out of attempts of other people, often people of authority in their lives, to "take them over." In the extreme, such attempts have resulted in physical or psychological abuse. Another form of damage can be inflicted by responding to youth as if the only thing that matters is their behavior. Concern for their inner confusion is missing altogether. Again, one of the tasks of pastoral care is to find that delicate balance between seeking to influence and attempting to control, helping a person find ways to exercise self-control and be a good steward of life, out of regard for himself or herself and others.

A Special Word about Teenage Pregnancy

Of course, one of the greatest fears of both parents of teenagers and teenagers themselves is that of pregnancy. The fear is sometimes expressed in ways that do not make sense to us, for example, by believing that safe sex "simply" means "control" of ejaculation or choosing the "safe" time of the month, or by believing that "just this one time" it won't happen. As in so many other cases, fears dealt with in distorted fashion become self-fulfilling prophecies.

In any case, when those occasions come—and they will—that a decision must be made because of pregnancy, the factors discussed already become even more important. It is true, on the one hand, that time is of the essence. On the other hand, it is also important to respect the need for time to acknowledge feelings and deeper issues—and to face choices.

Pregnancy is made all the more difficult for teenagers and their families because of the emotional intensity that surrounds the issue of abortion. Unfortunately, a pastor cannot somehow create a "safe harbor" unaffected by all the threats and political investments that a variety of people will have in the final decision. It is the hope of this author that any pastor will be self-aware enough and concerned enough about the *many* lives involved to avoid the dangers of falling into the role of an advocate for anyone other than the teenager struggling with the decision. Not only life, but also the quality of life, of mother, father, friends, and prospective child is involved. In the throes of a decision, the pregnant teenager needs to know of all the resources available, the known potential consequences of various choices, and, most of all, of the assurance that her pastor is *for her*, whatever she decides in this finite and painful moment in her life.

For Further Reading

Because this chapter is focused on a population group rather than a single issue, a more general bibliography is provided here. The reader will find that each of these works provides additional resources on the topics developed.

It is particularly important for a pastor to have a ready collection of books such as those listed here. Parents and teenagers are not likely to have such information available when a critical moment arises. Then, it is helpful to provide bibliotherapy as well as caring concern. Generally, a very helpful set of resources is to be found at any local chapter of Planned Parenthood. Contrary to the beliefs of many, this organization is an unusually rich resource for both literature and programs on responsible teenage sexuality.

Adams, Caren, Jennifer Fay, and Jan Loreen-Martin. *No Is Not Enough: Helping Teenagers Avoid Sexual Assault*. San Luis Obispo, Calif.: Impact Publishers, 1988.

Barnard, Charles P., ed. *Families, Incest, and Therapy: A Special Issue of the International Journal of Family Therapy*. New York: Human Sciences Press, 1983.

Blume, Judy. *Letters to Judy: What Your Kids Wish They Could Tell You*. New York: G. P. Putnam's Sons, 1986.

Calderone, Mary S., and James W. Ramey. *The Family Book about Sexuality*. San Francisco: Harper & Row, 1989.

Crooks, Robert, and Karla Baur. *Our Sexuality*, 4th ed. Redwood City, Calif.: Benjamin/Cummings, 1990.

Fortune, Marie. *Sexual Abuse Prevention: A Study for Teenagers*. Cleveland, Ohio: Pilgrim Press, 1984.

————. *Sexual Violence: The Unmentionable Sin*. New York: Pilgrim Press, 1983.

Goodwin, Norma J., ed. *Black Adolescent Pregnancy: Prevention and Management*. New York: Human Sciences Press, 1986.

Gordon, Sol, and Judith Gordon. *Raising a Child Conservatively in a Sexually Permissive World*. Rev. ed. New York: Fireside Books/Simon & Schuster, 1989.

Group for the Advancement of Psychiatry. *Crises of Adolescence:. Teenage Pregnancy, Impact on Adolescent Development*. New York: Brunner/Mazel, 1986.

Henshaw, S. K., A. M. Kenney, D. Somberg, and J. Van Vort. *Teenage Pregnancy in the United States: The Scope of the Problem and State Responses*. New York: Alan Guttmacher Institute, 1989.

Hyde, Margaret. *Teen Sex*. Philadelphia: Westminster Press, 1988.

Kaplan, Helen Singer. *Making Sense of Sex: The New Facts about Sex and Love for Young People*. New York: Simon & Schuster, 1979.

Presbyterian Church (U.S.A.). *God's Gift of Sexuality*. Louisville, Ky.: Presbyterian Publishing House, 1989.

Wattleton, Faye, and Elisabeth Kieffer. *How to Talk to Your Child about Sexuality*. New York: Doubleday, 1986.

8
Homosexuality

After rescheduling their appointment with their pastor three times, Mel and Joyce finally appeared. They looked sad and tired. After a few minutes of half-hearted attempts at general conversation and comments on the weather punctuated by silence, the minister observed that they seemed deeply troubled about something. With a sigh, Mel looked up and said, "I don't know what to say or do. So, I might just as well say it. Our son told us three weeks ago that he is gay. We haven't slept a full night since. What are we going to do?" Then Joyce interjected, "I don't worry so much about what we are going to do as I wonder about what we must have done to make him turn out like that."

The Theological

The issue of homosexuality is volatile—laced with grief and hope, anger and frustration. Not only are there powerful emotions, but there are strong and conflicting theological views based on widely divergent interpretations of scripture. Interestingly enough, supporters and critics of homosexual orientation as a valid Christian lifestyle center their arguments on the same passages of scripture rather than seeking out texts that seem to dispute each other. Here are just a few examples.

In Genesis 19, when a crowd demands that Lot send out his guests (two strangers, called angels in the text) so that the crowd may "know" them, Lot attempts to send his daughters out to the crowd instead. The crowd refuses Lot's attempt to protect the visitors in the shelter of his home, and they threaten to harm Lot

127

and his family as well. As a result of the crowd's actions, the angels/guests announce that they will destroy Sodom for its wickedness. The question that is argued among the debaters of homosexuality, of course, revolves around what evil the angels and God had in mind when deciding to destroy the city. One school of thought asserts that the sin of Sodom was its citizens' "obvious" attempt at homosexual rape of the guest angels/strangers. Another point of view, based on the customs of the time, interprets the text to mean that the sin was one of inhospitality to strangers. Still others point out that Lot himself was offering his own daughters to be "gang-raped," a heterosexual act, which he may have thought the crowd wanted. Yet another interpretation takes the story as one of many examples in which a general condemnation is being made of any behavior that inflicts abusive, lustful, or demeaning acts upon anyone. Each of these perspectives seeks to identify a specific crime or crimes being condemned by God.

A similar array of perspectives revolves around the passages of Leviticus 18:22 and 20:13. Both verses refer to a male "lying with another male as with a woman." Is this a universal condemnation of homosexuality? One side would say, "Of course! The text is quite clear on the matter." Another side would say, "No. This is another case in which a particular example of abusive or demeaning behavior is being condemned." Still others would simply note that the laws in Leviticus also prohibit eating rare meat, harvesting all the grain in a field, and touching a woman who is menstruating. They are simply not literally applicable to Christians without careful analysis of their context within the life of ancient Israel.

The text that all sides seem to agree is most crucial is Romans 1:26–27. Paul refers there to men and women giving up natural intercourse for unnatural. Immediately the proponents of homosexuality as a sin note the condemnation. Others point out that the context here is idolatry, and that homosexual activity, as a runaway passion, is indeed sinful—as is any other passion that turns one away from God. Further, some scholars point out that the issue of pederasty may well have been the concern being addressed in this text, as is the case in 1 Corinthians 6:9.

So, the debate goes on. All sides of the debate do admit that the matter of homosexual *orientation* is not addressed directly in scripture. However, says one side, if the act is condemned, then the orientation is condemned by implication. Others would say, "No! There is a big difference between orientation and acts." The condemnation of particular acts is based on the motives of the initiator and the impact of the actions on the other person. For example, a slap on the back, depending on all sorts of variables, may be experienced as a friendly gesture by one recipient or an act of aggression by another. And the motivation of the person doing the slapping must be analyzed as well. Such is the case with homosexual behavior.

Of course there are more than just two theological points of view in the current debate about homosexuality. One is a view that concerns itself primarily with sin. Within that sin-focused camp there are differences over whether the sin is located in behavior only or whether even the preference, acted out or not, is sinful. Or, again, is sin involved only if children or nonconsenting adults are involved?

Another point of view shifts the emphasis from sin to finitude. This outlook holds that homosexual orientation and activity may well reflect "arrested development," a term that emerges from psychoanalytic literature and is appropriated by theologians as an example of human limitations caused by nature or nurture. Within this range of perspective based on an understanding of human finitude, homosexual orientation is understood as an expression of life that falls short of the "norm" that God intended for humankind. Homosexual orientation, then, might be compared to genetic defects or some form of disability in which a person, for physical, mental, or psychological reasons not of his or her own choosing, will fail to experience the fullness of human life.

At the other end of the continuum is a perspective that life, as God created it, is rich and varied. Just as there are different skin colors, body shapes, and expressions of intelligence and creativity, so there are different sexual orientations and preferences. A minority race is not seen as inferior or of less value or acceptability than a majority. Neither should such assumptions be made about a minority group in terms of sexual orientation. All these groups, majorities and minorities, are called to live according to an ethic that opposes abusive, demeaning, or lustful acts imposed on others.

In the midst of these differences, it is also important to be aware of the points of unity that exist in the debate. The shared perspective seems to be that *all* persons, regardless of sexual orientation, are children of God and thus deserving recipients of God's grace. Therefore, we are called upon to view persons of homosexual orientation with the same regard in which we hold all people. Supportive and caring relationships should be offered, and all people are to be welcomed into the life and work of the church.

Of course, our motives for extending care will vary according to the view held with regard to the homosexual issue. One welcome will be extended as part of a call to repentance, with the promise of prayer and support for those struggling to overcome the "sin" of homosexual preference and/or activity. A welcome from another point of view will be accompanied by the promise of sustaining ministry, acknowledging the likelihood that a change of orientation is not possible. Within those limits on the possibility of change, coping mechanisms will be taught and encouraged, with welcome into the fellowship of the church always assured. In the third case, affirmation of homosexual orientation will be given—accompanied by encouragement to express that orientation with the same concern for monogamy and faithfulness that is expected of heterosexual relationships.

Much more can be said, and is said vociferously, about these divergent viewpoints. It is important for a pastor to be aware of them and to be working toward some articulate stance for himself or herself with regard to them. However, it is not the purpose of this book to provide a full development of the perspectives here. Bibliographical suggestions are provided at the end of this chapter for the reader who wishes to explore them further.

Within this diversity of theological opinion, there is always a place for pastoral care, and we shall focus on suggestions for care and support later in this chapter. The form of care expressed to Joyce and Mel, the couple introduced at the beginning of this chapter, will be influenced by the theological viewpoint of the pastor. But that viewpoint alone should not be the final determining factor.

The Psychological

As in the theological realm, there is debate among and within psychological circles about the origins and normality of homosexual orientation. Certainly there is mutually shared concern and outrage about victimizing persons, adult or child, by sexual seduction or rape. However, in cases of mutual consent between adults, it is increasingly the view that therapeutic intervention is appropriate only at the request of one or both parties.

The *Diagnostic and Statistical Manual of Mental Disorders*, Third Edition—Revised (Washington, D.C.: American Psychiatric Association, 1987), hereafter referred to as DSM-III-R, is an official publication of the American Psychiatric Association. It organizes and describes currently accepted diagnoses of human emotional problems considered to be disorders in need of treatment. It also provides the common and current language by which these disorders are professionally described and understood. That book's own definition of a mental disorder is helpful to our present discussion.

> In DSM-III-R each of the mental disorders is conceptualized as a clinically significant behavior or psychological syndrome or pattern that occurs in a person and that is associated with present distress (a painful symptom) or disability (impairment

in one or more important areas of functioning) or with a significantly increased risk of suffering death, pain, disability, or an important loss of freedom. In addition, this syndrome or pattern must not be merely an expectable response to a particular event, e.g., the death of a loved one. Whatever its original cause, it must currently be considered a manifestation of a behavioral, psychological, or biological dysfunction in the person. Neither deviant behavior, e.g., political, religious, or sexual, nor conflicts that are primarily between the individual and society are mental disorders unless the deviance or conflict is a symptom of a dysfunction in the person, as described above. (DSM-III-R, p. xxii)

Within the parameters of this definition, homosexual orientation does not qualify as a disorder. From the vantage point of DSM-III-R it is not a manifestation of "dysfunction." Some would say that it is a kind of unacceptable "deviant behavior" from a number of religious, sexual, or political perspectives, but, as noted in the definition above, such a characteristic does not qualify it as an emotional or mental disorder, or as a "sickness."

Note the last sentence in the definition above. It is a reminder that mental diagnosis has been used in some times and places as a means of control. This refusal in DSM-III-R to diagnose homosexual orientation as a disorder gives expression to the resistance among many mental health professionals to their profession being used as a means to enforce standards of behavior. Though the wording is complex, it is helpful to become familiar with the language and concepts reflected here.

One additional illustration from DSM-III-R may be helpful. One chapter in the manual is titled "Sexual Disorders." The disorders in that section are divided into two groups. The paraphilias are a group that includes "arousal in response to sexual objects or situations" that are not part of the "normal" arousal patterns for people. These paraphiliac disorders also "interfere with the capacity for reciprocal affectionate sexual activity." The second group is called the sexual dysfunctions, and they comprise the patterns that inhibit sexual desire, as well as psychological and physiological changes that interfere with normal sexual response (DSM-III-R, p. 279).

Note that both of these two major groups have to do with *inappropriate objects* of sexual stimulation or *inhibition* of sexual desire. Neither of those two categories are amenable to the inclusion of homosexual orientation. The only reference to homosexuality in DSM-III-R is found in a classification titled "Sexual Disorder Not Otherwise Specified." Within that general classification, one example is "persistent and marked distress about one's sexual orientation" (p. 296). Here, however, the disorder is not homosexuality (or heterosexuality) as such. Rather, it has to do with persistent distress *about* one's orientation.

Homosexuality was included, years ago, in the classification of emotional and mental disorders. However, after great debate (which still goes on in some quarters), it was dropped from the official classification system.

Within the official world of psychiatry and psychology, then, homosexuality in and of itself is not viewed as a disorder. Treatment and attention are available, however, to help someone with the adjustment to homosexual orientation in the midst of a culture or subculture that condemns such orientation and behavior.

Despite the absence of homosexuality as a disorder in DSM-III-R, there are points of view within the psychological community that do see it as a developmental disorder. The term often used is "arrested development," referred to earlier in our theological discussion. Implied in the use of the label is the belief that normal development in human beings progresses toward heterosexual orientation, which is viewed as "mature." While a mature adult is capable of loving both males and females, one's preference in a specifically sexual, or genital, relationship will be tipped in favor of the gender other than one's own.

Developmental theorists and clinicians all agree that it is normal within the human growth cycle to move through a period of fascination with, and often experimentation with, partners of the same sex. Harry Stack Sullivan, a well-known writer on psychiatry, relationships, and human development earlier in this century, described this period of prepuberty as the "chumship era."

Disagreements occur around what happens next. The advocates of the view that homosexual orientation is arrested development maintain that after having found comfort in and security with one's own gender identity, a normally maturing person then moves into puberty and adolescence with a disposition toward a shift in primary affection toward the other gender. When development is arrested, that shift does not take place. Opinions within this camp then differ over causes and whether attempts to overcome this condition can be successful.

Proponents of homosexual orientation as one of several normal developmental outcomes, of course, argue that attempts to change one's homosexual preference are attempts to change the structure of one's personality. Therefore, they are inappropriate. Divergent opinion occurs again over whether that basic orientation is "set" by environmental or biological factors, or by both.

Environmental or psychological influences that some believe may shape one's sexual orientation include psychological and physical trauma, satisfying and painful relationships, intensely voiced and enforced moral codes, and more. One of the earlier theories about psychological influences that could result in homosexual orientation was that of the strong mother and the passive father. However, a number of recent studies have demonstrated that no clearly documentable and predictable connection can be made between such a parental constellation and homosexual orientation.

Continuing genetic research is taking place with regard to sexual orientation. Some researchers are referring to a person who seems to be homosexually oriented as a result of psychological influences and choices as having "secondary" homosexual orientation. "Primary" orientation is understood to have biological roots and will be discussed in the next section.

With the exception of a strong vocal minority, the clinical disciplines generally view attempts to change a person's sexual orientation as extremely difficult, if not impossible. Therapeutic energy tends to be devoted to supporting one's acceptance of that orientation if it is troubling, and to the design of a lifestyle that can be both fulfilling and not dangerous to the self or others.

The Biological

Two different and important biological issues should be noted. The first, though not fully verified, is the conviction of an increasing number of medical scientists that the roots of primary homosexual orientation lie not in psychological or cultural roots but in biochemical or genetic ones. General confirmation of such a view will raise a number of fascinating and, for some, troubling issues. Sexual orientation will be understood as a genetic predisposition, as are many temperamental characteristics and propensities toward particular diseases. Such predispositions are understood to be "set" prior to birth. Environmental influences only play a part in affecting the relative comfort or discomfort within which that orientation is lived out, rather than in determining or reshaping the orientation itself.

Tied to the impact of sexual hormones on the fetus during pregnancy, the process by which this genetic shaping is thought to take place is far too complex to be explored in this discussion. Needless to say, these ongoing studies will have a strong impact on current psychological and therapeutic perspectives, and will call for careful theological reflection as well.

The second biological issue to be noted is that of sexually transmitted diseases (STDs). The connections drawn between homosexuality and AIDS (acquired immunodeficiency syndrome) have received much attention in the press. While it is incorrect to draw an exclusive line of cause and effect between homosexuality and AIDS, anyone involved in homosexual activity needs to be acutely conscious of the fact that passage of the disease from one person to another is accomplished through the exchange of bodily fluids. Unprotected penetration, ejaculation, and/or bleeding in another person's body cavities occur frequently in both homosexual and heterosexual relations. Anal intercourse is particularly risky because of the thin wall of the rectum. The AIDS threat exists, also, through exchanging needles among drug addicts.

Pastoral Strategy

With all the above information circulating inside the pastor's head, the question of extending care to Mel and Joyce returns to the fore. And Mel and Joyce are not unique. Theirs is only one of the array of homosexual issues that can be brought to a pastor. Other possibilities include: a teenager struggling with the fear that he or she is homosexual; a college student or young adult struggling with how to tell her or his parents of a chosen homosexual lifestyle; a troubled spouse coming to acknowledge homosexual orientation and asking what to do about a marriage to a loving heterosexual partner; a troubled spouse who has discovered that his or her partner is gay or lesbian; an officer in a congregation who is gay and wants to know whether to resign his position; a member of a congregation who is asking for use of the church for a support group for homosexuals; parents who are troubled by the discovery that their child's fourth-grade teacher is lesbian. Regardless of the agenda and circumstances that have brought you and any of these people together, there are some very basic approaches that will be important.

Some Pastoral Events

In that first visit, Mel and Joyce talked about their fears and sense of guilt for an hour or so. At the conclusion of the conversation, they were emotionally fatigued, but they also looked relieved. "I just needed to *say it* to somebody," said Mel. "I needed you to talk it out with someone other than me," said Joyce with a tired smile on her face. "But," they both then asked, "what do we do now?"

Their pastor's suggestion was that they come back again after having talked with each other about what they wanted to know, about homosexuality in general and about their son in particular. Some general reading about homosexuality was also suggested. Part of the agreement was that they would not *do* anything in the interim, unless an emergency arose. The suggestion to continue talking with each other about what they wanted to know was a way of helping them continue to rely on their own close bonds with each other. A subtle shift was being suggested as well. Now, instead of only worrying out loud with each other, they were focusing on a plan and finding their points of common concern and interest. Cognitive dimensions were being added to their already taxed emotional involvement. Spiritual and theological concerns were to be discerned as well.

When they returned ten days later, they had a long list of topics. The result was a discussion, accompanied by more specific suggestions for reading material, that led to further feelings of fascination and relief. As they learned more, they became eager to talk with their son again. Up until that point they had been avoiding anything other than the most superficial conversations with him.

As they shared their interest and curiosity about homosexuality with their son, he gratefully began to talk to them with less defensiveness. Over time, without any decisions being made, they began to communicate with each other in ways that had not occurred for several years. Ultimately, working through a few occasions of tension, they built a relationship in which they could express their fears without taking an unnecessary stand over and against him. He could continue to be in touch with them without demanding some sort of "endorsement" or setting himself up for rejection. It was a far better outcome than they had imagined possible.

In another pastoral situation altogether, the minister was visited by a woman in her forties who revealed her long-term lesbian relationship with her roommate of fifteen years. The impetus for this visit was the news just received that her mother was terminally ill. Neither of her parents knew (she thought!) of her homosexuality, and she felt guilty about keeping such a secret from them. Now, she wanted to know whether or not to tell them.

It was an agenda of "getting things in order" for death. Before her mother's death, she wanted to break through the barrier created by her secret. "But," she said, recognizing the irony of her words, "I'm afraid it would kill her."

Over the next three weeks, this gutsy woman met with the pastor several times to "rehearse" her conversation with her parents. She read material about communication, problem solving, conflict resolution, and anything else she could get her hands on. Hopes and fears, interlaced with new ideas for how to "manage" the conversation, were voiced. Finally, she was ready. Although the pastor offered to accompany her, she decided to go it alone.

The next day she called with choked voice to say that she told her story sitting on the bed holding her mother's hand, with her father sitting in a chair close by. "The miracle," she said, "was that they *knew*! And they had loved me enough not to ask until I let them know that I was ready. Why didn't I do this sooner?" Her question was not one of bitterness, but of relief and gratitude.

The two examples above were both situations in which the pastor could work with the people all the way through to some resolution of the issues. The major needs were for a safe and confidential place to explore, a source for information, an opportunity to "test out" decisions, and a place to return to celebrate and/or grieve over the outcomes of action taken.

There are situations, of course, in which the pastor will not be equipped professionally or will not have the time. An example is the situation of a person who wants to confront directly his or her own homosexual orientation. Such was the case with Jonathan, a young man of twenty-three, who came to his pastor's study.

Jonathan was direct and to the point. "I am a homosexual," he said. "And I don't want to be." He then went on to describe a series of unhappy relationships with women through his teen years. While he enjoyed their company, he rarely had become sexually aroused. Serious relationships had ended when the women discovered his lack of responsiveness and backed off, saying he was "weird."

In college he had developed two different gay relationships, both of which had lasted for some time. Both had been broken off by him. Frightened by his enjoyment of and attraction to those partners, he had spent the last year of college in a very reclusive existence. Now, having graduated, he wanted to confront the issue head on.

The pastor recognized that this therapeutic and spiritual journey would be a long one, and no promises could be made about the outcome. He and Jonathan had several lengthy conversations about homosexuality, including several theological and psychological points of view. The desire of this young man remained to move into treatment. Referral was made, and pastoral contact was maintained.

Should you need to make a referral, use the general principles outlined in chapter 3. In addition, inquire of the people to whom you refer about his or her attitude toward homosexuality both personally and professionally. Be sure the person is reasonably comfortable with and supportive of persons wrestling with issues of sexual preference. Do not settle for someone who treats anybody, regardless of the issue. Make sure that the person has experience and training in dealing with *this* issue. Again, referral suggestions from a university hospital department of psychiatry can be quite helpful. The major pastoral responsibility is to help parishioners get to professional people who are competent and caring.

Conclusion

Of course, the examples given above are relatively positive in their outcomes. Surely there are negative ones. The point here, however, is that a pastor can provide a context within which the odds can at least be in favor of reconciliation and caring.

In all these cases, the pastoral relationship served as a safe place within which "rehearsal" could take place for confronting difficult situations. Through the provision of gentle and patient listening, followed by invitations to learn more and to work to assure the best possible outcomes, relationships were preserved and strengthened. *That* should be the pastoral task, rather than rendering a judgment on things that probably cannot be changed.

Surely there are times and places in the work of ministry when strong stands must be taken and corrective words might well be spoken. This is not one of them. Homosexuality has so many unknowns, and feelings are so strong, that some place is needed within which to explore and understand and remain connected—even as God remains faithful to us by offering such gifts.

For Further Reading

Because of the emotional intensity generated by homosexuality, a flood of literature is on the market. The attempt here is to provide a balanced bibliography to enable the interested reader to find articulate arguments for a variety of perspectives. The list is divided between specifically pastoral/theological literature and the work of a number of writers in the sciences.

Pastoral/Theological Literature

Barnhouse, Ruth Tiffany. *Homosexuality: A Symbolic Confusion.* San Francisco: Seabury Press, 1979.

Barnhouse, Ruth Tiffany, and Urban T. Holmes III. *Male and Female: Christian Approaches to Sexuality.* San Francisco: Seabury Press, 1976.

Boswell, John. *Christianity, Social Tolerance, and Homosexuality.* Chicago: University of Chicago Press, 1980.

Cobb, John. *Matters of Life and Death.* Louisville, Ky.: Westminster/John Knox Press, 1991.

Consiglio, William. *Homosexual No More.* Wheaton, Ill.: Victor Books, 1991.

Countryman, William. *Dirt, Greed, and Sex.* Minneapolis: Fortress Press, 1988.

Edwards, George R. *Gay/Lesbian Liberation: A Biblical Perspective.* New York: Pilgrim Press, 1984.

Furnish, Victor. *The Moral Teachings of Paul,* 2d ed. Nashville: Abingdon Press, 1985.

Gramick, Jeannine, ed. *Homosexuality in the Priesthood and the Religious Life.* New York: Crossroad Publishing Co., 1969.

Horner, Thomas M. *Jonathan Loved David: Homosexuality in Biblical Times*. Philadelphia: Westminster Press, 1978.

McNeill, John J. *The Church and the Homosexual*. Kansas City: Sheed, Andrews & McMeel, 1976.

Mickey, Paul A. *Of Sacred Worth*. Nashville: Abingdon Press, 1991.

Nelson, James B. *The Intimate Connection: Male Sexuality, Masculine Spirituality*. Philadelphia: Westminster Press, 1988.

Oberholtzer, W. Dwight, ed. *Is Gay Good? Ethics, Theology, and Homosexuality*. Philadelphia: Westminster Press, 1971.

Scanzoni, Letha, and Virginia Ramey Mollenkott. *Is the Homosexual My Neighbor? Another Christian View*. San Francisco: Harper & Row, 1978.

Scroggs, Robin. *The New Testament and Homosexuality*. Philadelphia: Fortress Press, 1983.

Switzer, David K., and Shirley Switzer. *Parents of the Homosexual*. Philadelphia: Westminster Press, 1980.

Wegner, Judith Romney. "Leviticus." In *The Women's Bible Commentary*, ed. Carol A. Newsom and Sharon H. Ringe. Louisville, Ky.: Westminster/John Knox Press, 1992.

Yamamoto, J., ed. *The Crisis of Homosexuality*. Wheaton, Ill.: Christianity Today/Victor Books, 1990.

From the Human Sciences

Bell, Alan P. *Sexual Preference: Its Development in Men and Women*. Bloomington, Ind.: Indiana University Press, 1981.

Cowan, Thomas. *Gay Men and Women Who Enriched the World*. Boston: Mulvey Books, 1988.

Friedman, R. *Male Homosexuality*. New Haven, Conn.: Yale University Press, 1988.

Greenberg, D. *The Construction of Homosexuality*. Chicago: University of Chicago Press, 1988.

Harry, J. *Gay Children Grown Up: Gender Culture and Gender Deviance*. Westport, Conn.: Praeger Publishers, 1982.

Marmor, J., ed. *Homosexual Behavior: A Modern Reappraisal*. New York: Basic Books, 1980.

Masters, William H., and Virginia E. Johnson. *Homosexuality in Perspective*. New York: Little, Brown & Co., 1979.

Moberly, E. *Psychogenesis: The Early Development of Gender Identity*. New York: Routledge & Kegan Paul, 1983.

Final Reflections

Because of the complexity of our humanity, there is no end to the variety of ways in which we can confuse and be confused, hurt and be hurt, misunderstand and be misunderstood. The arena of sex and sexuality is a primary environment in which all these human foibles make themselves visible and felt. Of course, it is also true that the remarkable beauty of our humanity offers a variety of riches within the sexual dimensions of our lives as well. However, pastors seldom hear of the enjoyments. Hence, this book has focused on areas of pain that seem to present themselves more frequently to pastors and other caregivers in the life of the church.

I hope the reader will find the perspectives and suggestions discussed in this book to be of value in approaching these sexual issues as part of the larger scope of pastoral care. In the best of all worlds, genuine pastoral care will enable persons to speak more openly of the things they are afraid to confront and find choices where they have felt themselves to be powerless. While people may not find full resolution for their difficulties, at least they can have pastoral companions along the way. Then growth and understanding are more likely to occur in spite of anxiety and fear.

In order for a caregiver to contribute to change in perspective and coping styles, I offer several final recommendations.

First, *devise a reading program for yourself in the subject area of sex and sexuality*. Do not just concentrate on sex therapy. Diversify. Read some of the theological papers that have been published by your denomination—and others. Read some of the self-help books that are on the market to help people wrestle with their sexual hang-ups and worries. The purpose of such reading is not so much to keep in touch with what is going on in the field as to be sensitized to the power and shaping influence that sexuality has on daily life. The volume of popular literature reveals the incredible effort people put into trying to work out the things that block their relationships. It shows how much people really care about each other. In its own way, the volumes of literature in this area are a concrete testimony to the commitment that human beings have invested in order to make relationships work. Hope sells! I trust the bibliographies supplied throughout this book will help you along the way.

Second, *remind yourself regularly that sex can be humorous.* Certainly there are plenty of dirty jokes about sex. They reflect our discomfort and attempts to dehumanize it as a way of pretending that it does not matter. But another thing those jokes do is remind us of the fascinating ways these strangely varied human shapes and practices somehow find ways to seek and express affection. Try to remember the first thing you thought when you found out how people make babies. Let yourself laugh once in a while at what we have to overcome in order to be who we are. A sense of humor helps us to maintain perspective. The ability to chuckle (empathetically and gently, of course) in the midst of a tense pastoral conversation sometimes communicates a sense of comfort and assurance that "we can overcome."

Third, along with those chuckles, *continually remind yourself that sex is good.* In the face of the hurt and fear experienced by those who struggle with the issues discussed in this book, it is hard at times to see sex as anything other than a source of anxiety and pain. If we cave in to that viewpoint, we will lose our capacity to invite others into a new way of being. God intended sexuality for our own good, as a way of connecting and caring and growing. When we have a clear understanding of who we are, both limited and gifted, we can accept that good gift with responsibility and joy. Our sexuality is a means of grace through which we comfort and share and rejoice with each other in thousands of different ways as we live together in God's good creation.